GASTRIC SLEEVE BARIATRIC COOKBOOK

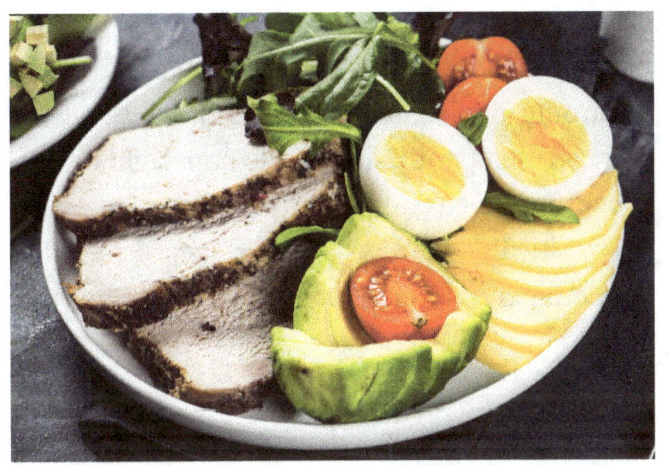

Elevate Your Post-Surgery Experience with Flavorful Recipes. A Culinary Collection to Empower Your Bariatric Success.

Dr. Jaclyn N. Anderson

Table of Contents

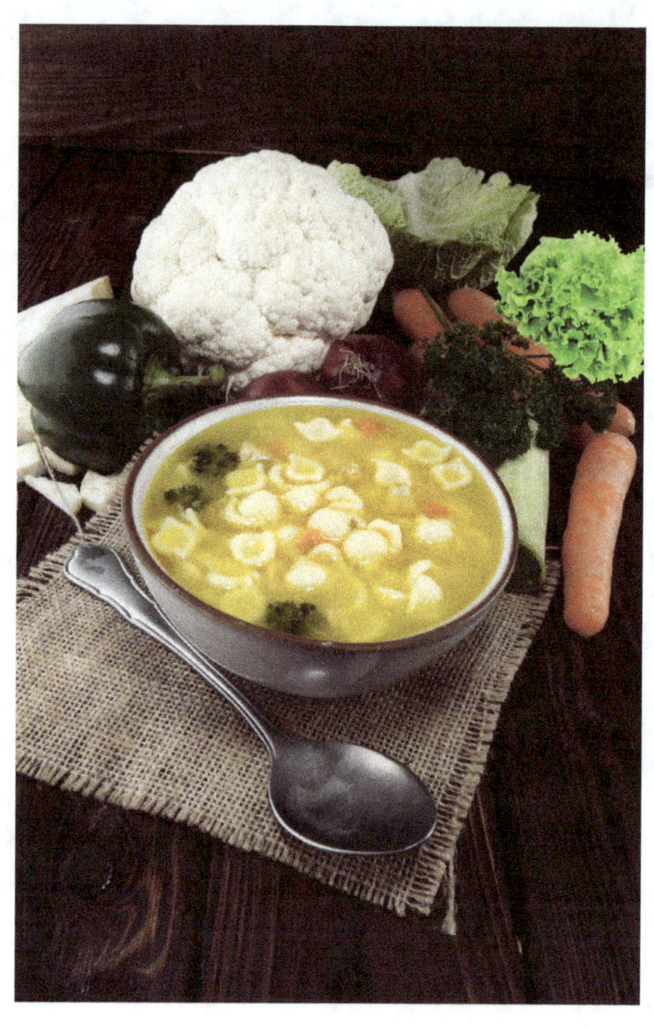

INTRODUCTION

Bariatric surgery, an increasingly prevalent solution for severe obesity, demands postoperative dietary adjustments crucial for a wholesome recovery. Following gastric sleeve surgery, altering eating habits becomes pivotal. This involves embracing smaller, more frequent meals with emphasis on protein and vital nutrients for hydration, while steering clear of sugary, fatty foods, carbonated drinks, and alcohol to avoid complications.

For those newly navigating life after gastric sleeve surgery, the implications are significant. It calls for careful food selection, ensuring adequate nutrient intake, and exploring new recipes that adhere to these dietary constraints. A specialized cookbook catering explicitly to gastric sleeve patients emerges as an invaluable tool, offering a balance between nutritional needs and flavorful diversity.

We've meticulously curated this Cookbook exclusively for you, housing a variety of breakfast, lunch, dinner, and snack recipes tailored to the specific dietary requirements of gastric sleeve patients. Moreover, it provides insights into optimizing your new dietary regimen for a seamless transition.

Each recipe within the Cookbook is thoughtfully outlined with easy-to-follow instructions and comprehensive nutritional breakdowns. Notably, these recipes prioritize low sugar, sodium, and fat content while being rich in protein and essential nutrients, often incorporating water-rich fruits and vegetables to support hydration—an essential element for post-operative gastric sleeve patients.

Whether you're seeking a quick breakfast fix or a fulfilling dinner that aligns with your dietary needs, this Cookbook offers the ideal recipe tailored for your recovery journey. Our aspiration is for these recipes not only to please your taste buds but also to serve as a guiding light in your pursuit of a healthy post-operative lifestyle. Say goodbye to dull, uninspiring, and unhealthy culinary choices!

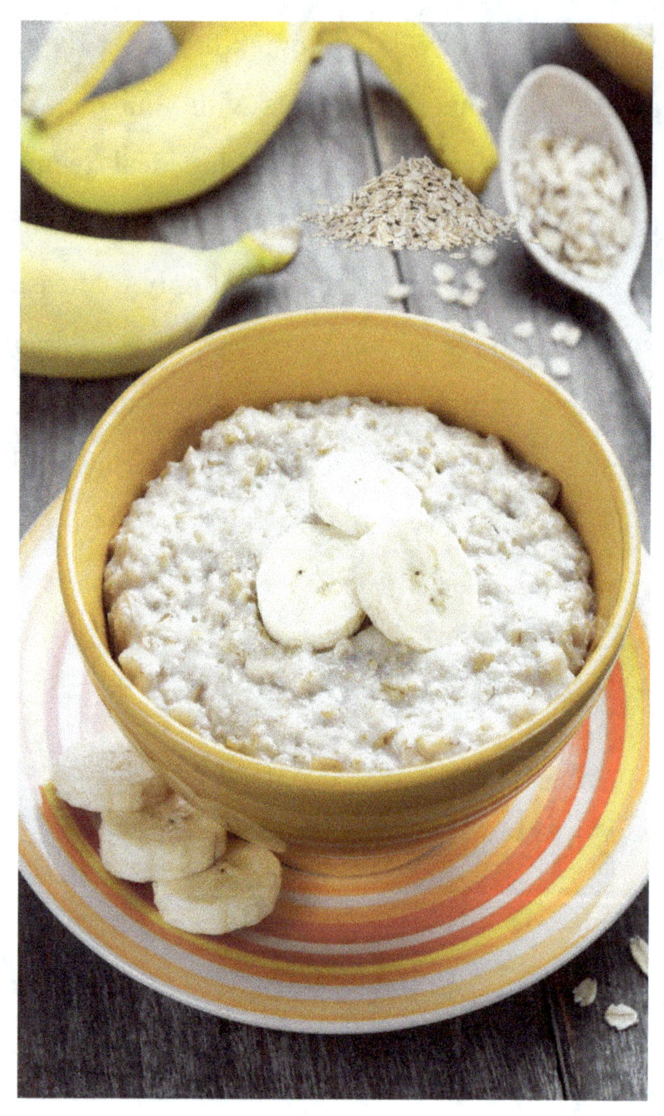

CHAPTER 1:

UNDERSTANDING GASTRIC SLEEVE SURGERY

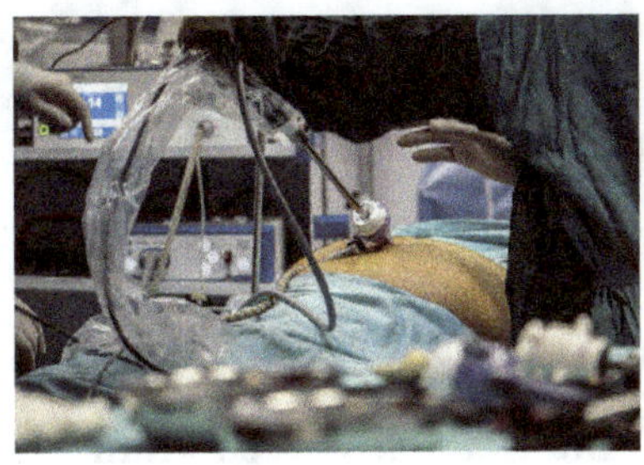

Gastric sleeve surgery, also known as sleeve gastrectomy, is a surgical procedure designed to assist with weight loss by reducing the stomach's size. This surgery is often recommended for individuals struggling with severe obesity, typically those with a body mass index (BMI) of 40 or higher, or 35 and higher with obesity-related health issues.

During the procedure, a surgeon removes a significant portion of the stomach, shaping it into a tube or sleeve-like structure. This reduction in stomach size restricts the amount of food it can hold, resulting in the patient feeling full more quickly and consuming fewer calories. Additionally, the surgery may alter gut hormones related to hunger and satiety, contributing to reduced appetite.

The surgery is usually conducted under general anesthesia and can often be performed using minimally invasive techniques, such as laparoscopy. This method involves making small incisions in the abdomen, inserting a camera and specialized surgical tools to carry out the procedure.

Post-surgery, patients are typically required to follow a strict diet and lifestyle changes to ensure a successful outcome. These modifications often involve consuming smaller meals, focusing on nutrient-dense foods, and avoiding high-calorie or sugary items. Moreover, regular exercise and ongoing medical monitoring are essential parts of the recovery and weight loss maintenance process.

As with any surgical procedure, gastric sleeve surgery carries potential risks and complications, including infection, blood clots, and, in rare cases, leaks from the surgical site. It's crucial for individuals considering this surgery to discuss the potential benefits and risks with a healthcare provider, who can provide personalized guidance based on the patient's health condition and history.

This surgery has demonstrated effectiveness in significant weight loss and improvement in weight-related health conditions, but it's essential to approach it as a part of a comprehensive weight management plan, including dietary changes, exercise, and long-term follow-up care for sustainable results.

Essential Nutritional Guidelines Post-Surgery

Following gastric sleeve surgery, it's crucial to adhere to a strict dietary plan to support your recovery and achieve the best results. Here are some essential nutritional guidelines for the post-surgery period:

1. **Clear Liquid Diet (First 1-2 Days):** In the immediate post-op period, you'll start with clear liquids only. This includes water, broth, sugar-free gelatin, and sugar-free clear juices. Sip these liquids slowly.

2. **Full Liquid Diet (Days 3-14):** Transition to full liquids like protein shakes, yogurt, and cream-based soups. These provide essential nutrients and protein to aid healing.

3. **Pureed Diet (Weeks 2-4):** Gradually introduce pureed foods such as mashed potatoes, cottage cheese, and blended lean meats. Make sure the texture is smooth.

4. **Soft Diet (Weeks 4-6):** Soft, easy-to-chew foods like scrambled eggs, cooked vegetables, and tender meats are appropriate. Avoid tough or fibrous foods.

5. **Regular Diet (After 6 Weeks):** Eventually, you can transition to a regular diet. Focus on lean proteins, fruits, vegetables, and whole grains. Continue to avoid high-sugar, high-fat, and high-calorie foods.

Nutritional Tips:

1. **Protein Intake:** Protein is crucial for healing and maintaining muscle mass. Aim for 60-80 grams of protein per day.

Consider lean meats, fish, poultry, tofu, and protein supplements if needed.

2. **Hydration:** Stay well-hydrated by sipping water throughout the day. Avoid carbonated and high-calorie beverages.

3. **Portion Control:** Your stomach is significantly smaller after surgery, so eat small, frequent meals. Listen to your body's signals of fullness.

4. **Vitamins and Supplements:** You may need to take vitamin and mineral supplements, especially vitamin B12, iron, calcium, and vitamin D, as nutrient absorption can be affected.

5. **Fiber:** Gradually introduce fiber-rich foods to prevent constipation, but avoid too much fiber in the early post-op period.

6. **Avoid High Sugar and High Fat Foods:** Sugary and fatty foods can lead to dumping syndrome, a group of

symptoms that can occur after consuming high-sugar or high-fat items.

7. **Slowly Reintroduce Foods:** When reintroducing new foods, monitor how your body reacts. Some foods may not be well-tolerated.

8. **Regular Follow-up:** Continue to meet with your healthcare team for regular check-ups and dietary guidance.

9. **Mindful Eating:** Pay attention to hunger and fullness cues. Eating slowly and savoring your meals can help prevent overeating.

Kitchen Tips for Gastric Sleeve Patients

1. **Invest in Smaller Utensils and Plates:** Using smaller plates and utensils can help control portion sizes, making it easier to manage smaller meals after surgery.

2. **Meal Prepping:** Plan and prepare meals in advance. Portion out food into smaller containers for easy access to appropriately sized meals throughout the week.

3. **Focus on Nutrient-Dense Foods:** Keep your kitchen stocked with nutrient-rich foods, such as lean proteins, fruits, vegetables, and whole grains. These will provide essential nutrients without excess calories.

4. **Prepare Soft and Blended Foods:** In the early stages after surgery, having soft and pureed foods ready can ease mealtime. Invest in a good blender to make smooth soups, purees, and blended meals.

5. **High-Protein Foods:** Ensure your kitchen has ample sources of high-quality protein, such as lean meats, fish,

eggs, Greek yogurt, and protein shakes or bars.

6. **Easy-to-Digest Snacks:** Keep easily digestible snacks on hand, like applesauce, low-fat cottage cheese, or low-sugar fruit cups for when you need a quick bite.

7. **Avoid Tempting Foods:** Keep high-calorie, high-sugar, and high-fat foods out of your kitchen to avoid temptation and to maintain a healthy eating environment.

8. **Label and Date Foods:** After preparing meals, label and date the containers to track freshness and avoid any spoilage.

9. **Experiment with Spices and Herbs:** Enhance the flavors of your meals with herbs and spices instead of heavy sauces or seasonings, which can be higher in calories.

10. **Create a Comfortable Eating Space:** Designate a comfortable and calming eating space in your kitchen to promote mindful eating without distractions.

11. **Stay Organized:** Keep your kitchen organized, with frequently used items within easy reach, making meal preparation and clean-up more efficient.

12. **Stay Hydrated:** Always have water easily accessible in your kitchen. Consider keeping a water bottle or jug nearby to encourage regular hydration.

13. **Small Kitchen Appliances:** Consider investing in small kitchen appliances like a food processor, blender, or air fryer to prepare healthy and easily digestible meals.

14. **Meal Planning Tools:** Use meal planning apps or whiteboards in your kitchen to schedule meals and keep track of your dietary intake.

15. **Support System:** Involve your family or support system in creating a conducive environment in the kitchen that aligns with your dietary needs and goals.

The Various Stages Involved In The Gastric Sleeve Process

Consultation and Evaluation:

- **Initial Consultation:** You meet with a bariatric surgeon to discuss your medical history, weight loss goals, and assess whether you're a suitable candidate for the surgery.

- **Evaluation:** Medical tests, including blood work, physical examinations, and sometimes psychological evaluations, are conducted to ensure you're physically and mentally prepared for the surgery.

Preparation Phase:

- **Education and Counseling:** Before the surgery, you'll receive guidance on the procedure, its risks, benefits, and the necessary lifestyle changes.

- **Pre-Surgery Diet:** You might be placed on a specific diet to reduce liver size and optimize safety for the surgery.

Surgery Day:

- **Anesthesia and Procedure:** The surgery is typically performed under general anesthesia. During the procedure, about 75-80% of the stomach is removed to create a sleeve-shaped stomach.

Immediate Post-Op Phase:

- **Hospital Stay:** You will spend a day or two in the hospital for monitoring. In some cases, patients may go home the same day if there are no complications.

- **Diet Progression:** Initially, you'll start with clear liquids, progressing through various diet stages as mentioned earlier.

Recovery and Follow-Up:

- **Physical Recovery:** The initial weeks involve healing and adapting to dietary changes. Patients gradually resume normal activities as directed by their healthcare team.

- **Follow-up Appointments:** Regular follow-up appointments with the surgeon and the dietitian to monitor progress, address concerns, and make necessary adjustments to the diet or medications.

Long-Term Management:

- **Diet and Lifestyle Changes:** Patients will need to maintain a modified diet and adhere to lifestyle changes to ensure weight loss and prevent complications.

- **Vitamin and Mineral Supplementation:** Long-term use of supplements may be recommended to prevent nutritional deficiencies due to reduced stomach capacity.

Insightful Advice For Every Step Of The Diet

1. Clear Liquid Phase:

Purpose: This phase helps in hydration and introduces easily digestible liquids.

Advice:

- Drink plenty of water to stay hydrated.
- Include clear broths, sugar-free gelatin, and non-caffeinated, sugar-free beverages.
- Sip slowly and avoid using straws as they can introduce excess air into the stomach, causing discomfort.

2. Full Liquid Phase:

Purpose: Introducing more nutrients and proteins while the stomach continues to heal.

Advice:

- Include protein shakes or smoothies without added sugar.

- Consume non-fat or low-fat dairy products like yogurt or milk.

- Blended soups and pureed vegetables can be included for added nutrition.

3. Semi-Solid Phase:

Purpose: Gradually introducing soft, easily digestible foods.

Advice:

- Incorporate foods like mashed potatoes, oatmeal, scrambled eggs, and well-cooked vegetables.

- Chew food thoroughly to a smooth consistency before swallowing.

- Avoid tough or fibrous foods that might be hard to digest.

4. Solid Phase:

Purpose: Gradual reintroduction of solid foods while being mindful of the stomach's reduced capacity.

Advice:

- Start with small portions and chew thoroughly.

- Focus on lean proteins, vegetables, and fruits.

- Avoid high-fat, high-sugar, or heavily processed foods.

- Take time to enjoy meals and stop eating when you feel full to prevent discomfort or nausea.

General Advice for all Phases:

1. **Chew Thoroughly:** Take your time to chew food well before swallowing, aiding in digestion and preventing discomfort.

2. **Stay Hydrated:** Drink water between meals to stay hydrated but avoid drinking

during meals to prevent overfilling the stomach.

3. **Follow Recommendations:** Adhere to your dietitian's guidelines and meal plans for the best results.

4. **Avoid Carbonated Beverages:** These can cause discomfort and bloat the stomach.

Foods To Consume And Avoid At Each Stage

1. Clear Liquid Phase:

Foods to Consume:

- Clear broths (vegetable, chicken, or beef)
- Sugar-free gelatin (jelly)
- Water
- Decaffeinated herbal tea
- Sugar-free, non-carbonated drinks

Foods to Avoid:

- Anything with pulp or solid pieces

- Dairy products

- Carbonated drinks

- Any beverages containing caffeine

- Sugary drinks or juices

2. Full Liquid Phase:

Foods to Consume:

- Protein shakes or smoothies without added sugar

- Unsweetened almond milk or low-fat dairy milk

- Unsweetened yogurt (low fat or Greek)

- Cream-based soups (strained or blended)

Foods to Avoid:

- Full-fat dairy products

- Smoothies with added sugars

- Carbonated beverages

- Drinks high in sugar or caffeine

3. Semi-Solid Phase:

Foods to Consume:

- Mashed potatoes

- Oatmeal

- Scrambled eggs or egg substitute
- Soft cooked vegetables (well-cooked)
- Canned fruits (in natural juices, no added sugar)

Foods to Avoid:

- Tough or fibrous foods
- Skins, seeds, or raw vegetables/fruits
- Spicy or heavily seasoned foods
- Large pieces of meat

4. Solid Phase:

Foods to Consume:

- Lean proteins (skinless poultry, fish, lean cuts of meat)
- Cooked vegetables and fruits
- Soft, easily chewable grains (quinoa, couscous)
- Small portions of nuts and seeds

Foods to Avoid:

- Tough or chewy meats
- Fibrous or stringy vegetables
- Foods high in sugar or fat

- Large meals in one sitting

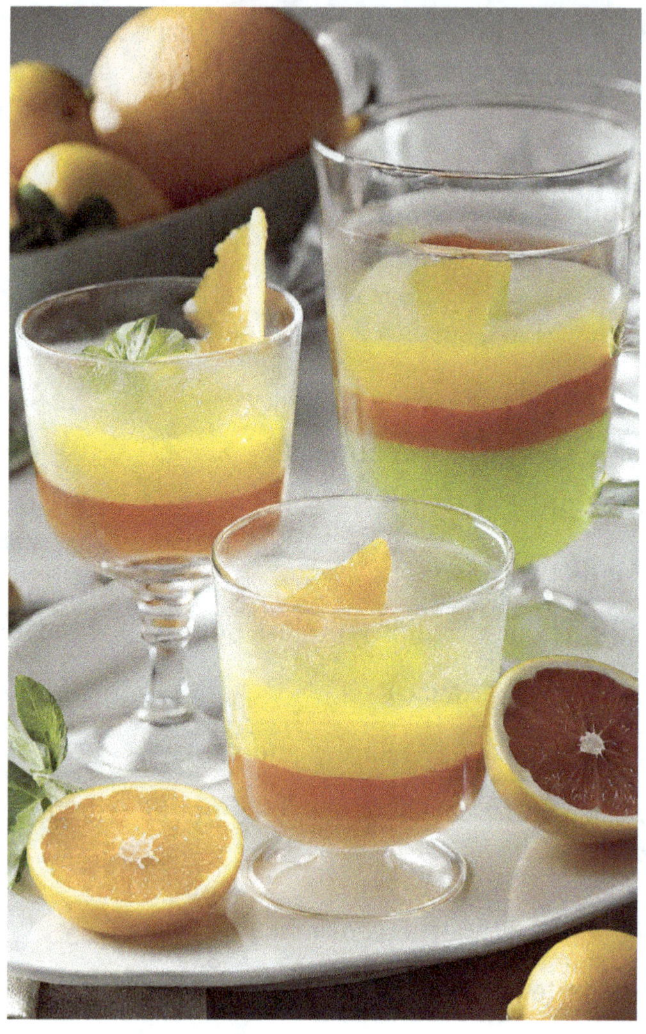

CHAPTER 2:

CLEAR LIQUID

Clear broths (vegetable, chicken, or beef)

Vegetable Clear Broth

Ingredients:

- 8 cups water
- 1 large onion, chopped
- 2 carrots, chopped
- 2 celery stalks, chopped
- 1 garlic clove, crushed
- 1 bay leaf
- Salt and pepper to taste

Nutritional Information (per serving):

Calories	Carbohydrates	Protein	Fat
15	4g	0.5g	0g

Preparation:

1. In a large pot, combine water, onion, carrots, celery, garlic, bay leaf, salt, and pepper.
2. Bring to a boil, then reduce heat and simmer for 45-60 minutes.
3. Strain the broth and discard the solids.

Chicken Clear Broth

Ingredients:

- 8 cups chicken broth (low sodium)
- 1 lb bone-in chicken parts (such as wings or thighs)
- 1 onion, chopped
- 2 carrots, chopped
- 2 celery stalks, chopped
- 2 sprigs fresh thyme
- Salt and pepper to taste

Nutritional Information (per serving):

Calories	Carbohydrates	Protein	Fat
40	4g	4g	1.5g

Preparation:

1. In a large pot, combine chicken broth, chicken parts, onion, carrots, celery, thyme, salt, and pepper.
2. Bring to a boil, then reduce heat and simmer for 45-60 minutes.
3. Remove the chicken parts, strain the broth, and discard the solids.

Beef Clear Broth

Ingredients:

- 8 cups beef broth (low sodium)
- 1 lb beef bones or oxtails
- 1 onion, chopped
- 2 carrots, chopped
- 2 celery stalks, chopped
- 2 cloves garlic, crushed

- 1 bay leaf
- Salt and pepper to taste

Nutritional Information (per serving):

Calories	Carbohydrates	Protein	Fat
50	2g	5g	2g

Preparation:

1. In a large pot, combine beef broth, beef bones or oxtails, onion, carrots, celery, garlic, bay leaf, salt, and pepper.
2. Bring to a boil, then reduce heat and simmer for 2-3 hours.
3. Remove the bones, strain the broth, and discard the solids.

Mushroom Clear Broth

Ingredients:

- 8 cups vegetable broth (low sodium)

- 1 lb assorted mushrooms (such as shiitake, cremini, or oyster), sliced
- 1 onion, chopped
- 2 cloves garlic, crushed
- 1-inch piece ginger, sliced
- 2-3 sprigs fresh thyme or parsley
- Salt and pepper to taste

Nutritional Information (per serving):

Calories	Carbohydrates	Protein	Fat
20	3g	2g	0.5g

Preparation:

1. In a pot, combine vegetable broth, mushrooms, onion, garlic, ginger, thyme or parsley, salt, and pepper.
2. Bring to a simmer and cook for 30-40 minutes.
3. Strain the broth, removing the solids.

Lentil Clear Broth

Ingredients:

- 8 cups water
- 1 cup dried green or red lentils
- 1 onion, chopped
- 2 carrots, chopped
- 2 celery stalks, chopped
- 2 cloves garlic, crushed
- 1 bay leaf
- Salt and pepper to taste

Nutritional Information (per serving):

Calories	Carbohydrates	Protein	Fat
35	7g	2g	0.2g

Preparation:

1. In a pot, combine water, lentils, onion, carrots, celery, garlic, bay leaf, salt, and pepper.

2. Bring to a boil, then reduce heat and
   simmer for 30-40 minutes until lentils
   are soft.

3. Remove the bay leaf and strain the broth.

Turkey Clear Broth

Ingredients:

- 8 cups turkey or chicken broth (low sodium)
- Turkey neck or wings
- 1 onion, chopped
- 2 carrots, chopped
- 2 celery stalks, chopped
- 2 sprigs fresh rosemary
- Salt and pepper to taste

Nutritional Information (per serving):

Calories	Carbohydrates	Protein	Fat
30	2g	3.5g	1.2g

Preparation:

1. In a pot, combine turkey or chicken broth, turkey parts, onion, carrots, celery, rosemary, salt, and pepper.

2. Bring to a simmer and cook for 45-60 minutes.

3. Remove the turkey parts, strain the broth, and discard solids.

Fish Clear Broth

Ingredients:

- 8 cups fish or seafood stock (low sodium)
- Fish bones or heads (non-oily fish)
- 1 onion, chopped
- 2 carrots, chopped
- 2 celery stalks, chopped
- 1 lemon, sliced
- Salt and pepper to taste

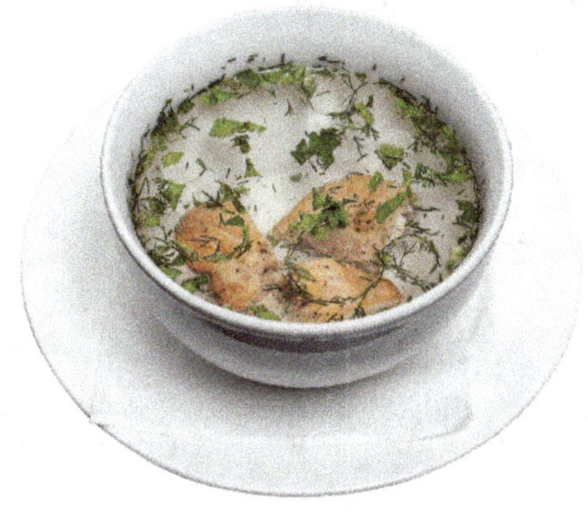

Nutritional Information (per serving):

Calories	Carbohydrates	Protein	Fat
25	3g	4g	0.5g

Preparation:

1. In a pot, combine fish or seafood stock, fish bones or heads, onion, carrots, celery, lemon, salt, and pepper.

2. Simmer for 30-45 minutes, skimming off any foam that forms on the surface.

3. Strain the broth to remove the solids.

Seaweed Clear Broth

Ingredients:

- 8 cups water

- 1 oz dried seaweed (kombu or wakame)

- 2 green onions, chopped

- 1-inch piece ginger, sliced

- 2 tablespoons low-sodium soy sauce

- Salt to taste

Nutritional Information (per serving):

Calories	Carbohydrates	Protein	Fat
10	2g	1g	0.1g

Preparation:

1. In a pot, combine water, seaweed, green onions, ginger, and soy sauce.

2. Bring to a simmer, then cook for 20-30 minutes.

3. Remove the seaweed, strain the broth, and discard solids.

Sugar-free gelatin (jelly)

Mixed Berry Gelatin

Ingredients:

- 2 cups mixed berries (strawberries, blueberries, raspberries)
- 1 packet sugar-free gelatin
- 2 cups boiling water

Nutritional Information (per serving):

Calories	Carbohydrates	Protein	Fat
15	2g	1g	0g

Preparation:

1. In a bowl, place the sugar-free gelatin. Pour boiling water over it and stir until dissolved.
2. Add mixed berries to the gelatin mixture.
3. Pour into molds or a shallow dish and refrigerate until set.

Citrus Medley Gelatin

Ingredients:

- Juice of 2 lemons and 2 limes
- Zest of 1 lemon and 1 lime
- 1 packet sugar-free gelatin
- 2 cups boiling water

Nutritional Information (per serving):

Calories	Carbohydrates	Protein	Fat
10	1.5g	1g	0g

Preparation:

1. In a bowl, combine sugar-free gelatin with boiling water, stirring until dissolved.

2. Add the citrus juice and zest to the gelatin mixture.

3. Pour into molds or a dish and refrigerate until set.

Peach Mango Gelatin

Ingredients:

- 1 cup pureed peaches and mangoes
- 1 packet sugar-free gelatin
- 2 cups boiling water

Nutritional Information (per serving):

Calories	Carbohydrates	Protein	Fat
20	3g	1g	0g

Preparation:

1. In a bowl, dissolve the sugar-free gelatin in boiling water.
2. Stir in the pureed peaches and mangoes.
3. Pour into molds or a dish and refrigerate until firm.

Apple Cinnamon Gelatin

Ingredients:

- 1 cup unsweetened applesauce
- 1 teaspoon cinnamon
- 1 packet sugar-free gelatin
- 2 cups boiling water

Nutritional Information (per serving):

Calories	Carbohydrates	Protein	Fat
15	3g	1g	0g

Preparation:

1. In a bowl, dissolve the sugar-free gelatin in boiling water.
2. Mix in the unsweetened applesauce and cinnamon.
3. Pour into molds or a dish and refrigerate until set.

Vanilla Coconut Gelatin

Ingredients:

- 1 cup unsweetened coconut milk

- 1 teaspoon vanilla extract
- 1 packet sugar-free gelatin
- 2 cups boiling water

Nutritional Information (per serving):

Calories	Carbohydrates	Protein	Fat
25	2g	1g	1.5g

Preparation:

1. Dissolve the sugar-free gelatin in boiling water in a bowl.
2. Mix in the unsweetened coconut milk and vanilla extract.
3. Pour into molds or a dish and refrigerate until firm.

Strawberry Kiwi Gelatin

Ingredients:

- 1 cup pureed strawberries and kiwi
- 1 packet sugar-free gelatin

- 2 cups boiling water

Nutritional Information (per serving):

Calories	Carbohydrates	Protein	Fat
15	2.5g	1g	0g

Preparation:

1. Dissolve the sugar-free gelatin in boiling water in a bowl.
2. Stir in the pureed strawberries and kiwi.
3. Pour into molds or a dish and refrigerate until set.

Cherry Almond Gelatin

Ingredients:

- 1 cup pureed cherries
- 1/2 teaspoon almond extract
- 1 packet sugar-free gelatin
- 2 cups boiling water

Nutritional Information (per serving):

Calories	Carbohydrates	Protein	Fat
20	3g	1g	0g

Preparation:

1. Dissolve the sugar-free gelatin in boiling water in a bowl.

2. Stir in the pureed cherries and almond extract.

3. Pour into molds or a dish and refrigerate until firm.

Decaffeinated herbal tea

Chamomile and Lavender Tea

Ingredients:

- 2 teaspoons dried chamomile flowers
- 1 teaspoon dried lavender
- 2 cups water

Nutritional Information (per serving):

Calories	Carbohydrates	Protein	Fat
0	0g	0g	0g

Preparation:

1. Boil the water in a pot.

2. Add the dried chamomile flowers and lavender to a teapot or a heatproof container.

3. Pour the boiling water over the herbs and let it steep for 5-7 minutes.

4. Strain and serve.

Ginger and Lemon Tea

Ingredients:

- 1-inch piece of fresh ginger, sliced

- Juice of half a lemon

- 2 cups water

Nutritional Information (per serving):

Calories	Carbohydrates	Protein	Fat
5	1g	0g	0g

Preparation:

1. Boil the water in a pot.

2. Add the sliced ginger to a teapot or heatproof container.

3. Pour the boiling water over the ginger, then add the lemon juice.

4. Let it steep for 5-7 minutes, strain, and serve.

Hibiscus and Rosehip Tea

Ingredients:

- 2 teaspoons dried hibiscus flowers
- 1 teaspoon dried rosehips
- 2 cups water

Nutritional Information (per serving):

Calories	Carbohydrates	Protein	Fat

5	1g	0g	0g

Preparation:

1. Boil the water in a pot.

2. Place the dried hibiscus flowers and rosehips in a teapot or heatproof container.

3. Pour the boiling water over the herbs and let it steep for 10-15 minutes.

4. Strain and serve.

Cinnamon and Turmeric Tea

Ingredients:

- 1 teaspoon ground cinnamon
- 1/2 teaspoon ground turmeric
- 2 cups water

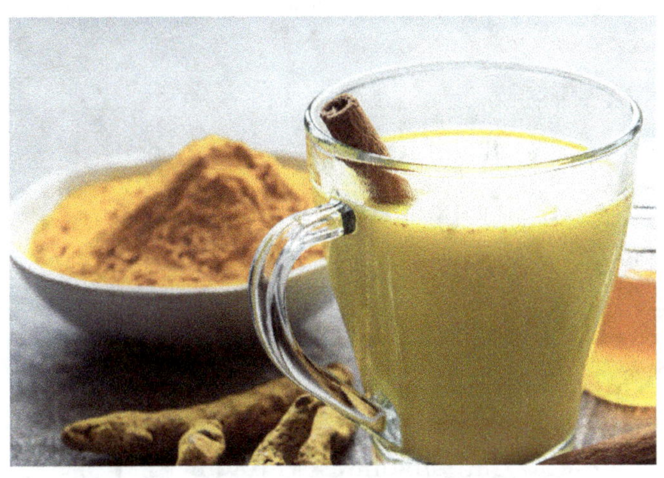

Nutritional Information (per serving):

Calories	Carbohydrates	Protein	Fat
5	1g	0g	0g

Preparation:

1. Boil the water in a pot.

2. Mix the ground cinnamon and turmeric in a teapot or heatproof container.

3. Pour the boiling water over the spices and let it steep for 5-7 minutes.

4. Strain and enjoy.

Lemongrass and Mint Tea

Ingredients:

- 2 stalks of lemongrass, crushed
- 1 tablespoon dried mint leaves
- 2 cups water

Nutritional Information (per serving):

Calories	Carbohydrates	Protein	Fat
0	0g	0g	0g

Preparation:

1. Boil the water in a pot.
2. Combine the crushed lemongrass and dried mint leaves in a teapot or heatproof container.
3. Pour the boiling water over the herbs and let it steep for 5-10 minutes.
4. Strain and serve.

Licorice Root and Fennel Seed Tea

Ingredients:

- 1 teaspoon licorice root
- 1 teaspoon fennel seeds
- 2 cups water

Nutritional Information (per serving):

Calories	Carbohydrates	Protein	Fat
5	1g	0g	0g

Preparation:

1. Boil the water in a pot.
2. Combine the licorice root and fennel seeds in a teapot or heat proof container.
3. Pour the boiling water over the ingredients and let it steep for 7-10 minutes.
4. Strain and enjoy.

Lemon Cucumber Infused Water

Ingredients:

- 4 cups water
- 1 lemon, thinly sliced
- 1/2 cucumber, thinly sliced

Nutritional Information (per serving):

Calories	Carbohydrates	Protein	Fat
0	0g	0g	0g

Preparation:

1. Combine water, lemon slices, and cucumber slices in a pitcher.
2. Chill in the refrigerator for a few hours to infuse flavors.
3. Serve over ice.

Berry Iced Tea

Ingredients:

- 2 cups brewed unsweetened tea, cooled

- 1/2 cup mixed berries (strawberries, blueberries, raspberries)

Nutritional Information (per serving):

Calories	Carbohydrates	Protein	Fat
5	1g	0g	0g

Preparation:

1. Blend the mixed berries until smooth.

2. Mix the berry puree with the brewed tea.

3. Serve over ice.

Pineapple Coconut Water

Ingredients:

- 3 cups coconut water

- 1/2 cup fresh pineapple chunks

Nutritional Information (per serving):

Calories	Carbohydrates	Protein	Fat
25	6g	1g	0g

Preparation:

1. Blend the fresh pineapple chunks until smooth.
2. Mix the pineapple puree with coconut water.
3. Serve chilled.

Watermelon Basil Cooler

Ingredients:

- 2 cups fresh watermelon chunks
- Handful of fresh basil leaves
- 2 cups water

Nutritional Information (per serving):

Calories	Carbohydrates	Protein	Fat
15	4g	1g	0g

Preparation:

1. Blend the watermelon chunks with water until smooth.
2. Add fresh basil leaves to the mixture and let it infuse for a few hours in the refrigerator.
3. Strain and serve over ice.

Minty Limeade

Ingredients:

- Juice of 4 limes
- Handful of fresh mint leaves
- 4 cups water

Nutritional Information (per serving):

Calories	Carbohydrates	Protein	Fat
10	3g	0g	0g

Preparation:

1. Mix lime juice and water in a pitcher.

2. Crush fresh mint leaves and add them to the limeade. Refrigerate for a few hours.

3. Strain and serve over ice.

Cranberry Hibiscus Punch

Ingredients:

- 2 cups unsweetened cranberry juice
- 1 tablespoon dried hibiscus flowers (steeped in 1/2 cup hot water, then cooled)
- 2 cups cold water

Nutritional Information (per serving):

Calories	Carbohydrates	Protein	Fat
20	5g	0g	0g

Preparation:

1. Steep the dried hibiscus flowers in hot water and let it cool.

2. Mix cranberry juice, hibiscus infusion, and cold water in a pitcher.

3. Serve over ice.

Mango Basil Sparkler

Ingredients:

- 1 cup fresh mango puree
- Handful of fresh basil leaves
- 3 cups sparkling water

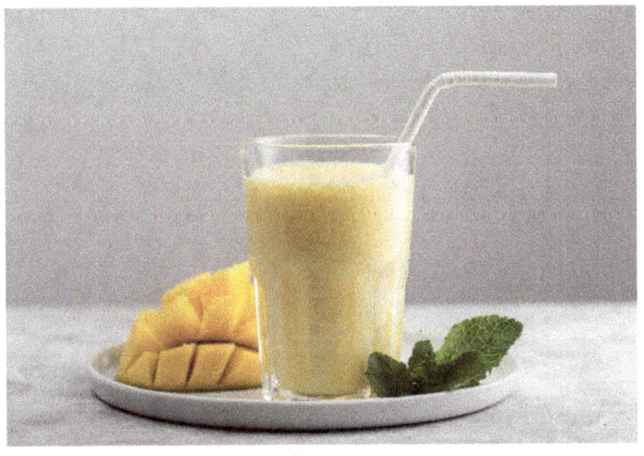

Nutritional Information (per serving):

Calories	Carbohydrates	Protein	Fat
30	8g	1g	0g

Preparation:

1. Blend the fresh mango into a puree.
2. Muddle basil leaves in a pitcher, add mango puree, and sparkling water.
3. Serve chilled.

CHAPTER 3:

FULL LIQUID PUREES

Protein Shakes Or Smoothies Without Added Sugar

Berry Blast Protein Smoothie

Ingredients:

- 1/2 cup mixed berries (strawberries, blueberries, raspberries)
- 1/2 cup plain Greek yogurt
- 1 scoop unflavored protein powder
- 1/2 cup unsweetened almond milk

Nutritional Information (approx. per serving):

Calories	Carbohydrates	Protein	Fat
150	10g	20g	3g

Preparation:

1. Blend mixed berries, Greek yogurt, protein powder, and almond milk until smooth.
2. Add more almond milk for desired consistency.

Peanut Butter Banana Protein Shake

Ingredients:

- 1 ripe banana
- 2 tablespoons natural peanut butter
- 1 scoop unflavored protein powder
- 1/2 cup unsweetened oat milk

Nutritional Information (approx. per serving):

Calories	Carbohydrates	Protein	Fat
280	30g	20g	10g

Preparation:

1. Blend banana, peanut butter, protein powder, and oat milk until well combined.

2. Add more milk for a thinner consistency.

Cocoa Banana Protein Smoothie

Ingredients:

- 1 ripe banana
- 1 tablespoon unsweetened cocoa powder
- 1 scoop unflavored protein powder
- 1/2 cup unsweetened soy milk

Nutritional Information (approx. per serving):

Calories	Carbohydrates	Protein	Fat
220	25g	20g	5g

Preparation:

1. Blend banana, cocoa powder, protein powder, and soy milk until creamy.

2. Increase or decrease the milk quantity for desired thickness.

Coconut Mango Protein Shake

Ingredients:

- 1/2 cup frozen mango chunks
- 1/2 cup unsweetened coconut milk
- 1 scoop unflavored protein powder
- 1 tablespoon shredded unsweetened coconut

Nutritional Information (approx. per serving):

Calories	Carbohydrates	Protein	Fat
230	20g	25g	8g

Preparation:

1. Blend frozen mango, coconut milk, protein powder, and shredded coconut until smooth.

2. Adjust the texture by adding more coconut milk if desired.

Chia Seed Strawberry Protein Smoothie

Ingredients:

- 1 cup fresh strawberries
- 1 tablespoon chia seeds
- 1 scoop unflavored protein powder
- 1/2 cup unsweetened almond milk

Nutritional Information (approx. per serving):

Calories	Carbohydrates	Protein	Fat
200	15g	20g	6g

Preparation:

1. Blend strawberries, chia seeds, protein powder, and almond milk until well combined.

2. Add more almond milk for a thinner consistency.

Pineapple Kiwi Protein Shake

Ingredients:

- 1/2 cup chopped fresh pineapple
- 1 kiwi, peeled and sliced
- 1 scoop unflavored protein powder
- 1/2 cup unsweetened coconut water

Nutritional Information (approx. per serving):

Calories	Carbohydrates	Protein	Fat
190	20g	20g	2g

Preparation:

1. Blend pineapple, kiwi, protein powder, and coconut water until smooth.
2. Adjust the thickness by adding more coconut water if needed.

Mocha Protein Shake

Ingredients:

- 1 cup cold brew coffee (unsweetened)
- 1 scoop unflavored or chocolate protein powder
- 1/2 cup unsweetened almond milk
- 1 tablespoon unsweetened cocoa powder

Nutritional Information (approx. per serving):

Calories	Carbohydrates	Protein	Fat
150	4g	25g	4g

Preparation:

1. Blend cold brew coffee, protein powder, almond milk, and cocoa powder until frothy.

2. Adjust thickness with more almond milk if desired.

Nutritious Yogurt Blend

Mixed Berry Yogurt Blend

Ingredients:

- 1/2 cup Greek yogurt
- 1/2 cup mixed berries (strawberries, blueberries, raspberries)
- 1 tablespoon honey (optional)
- 1 tablespoon chia seeds

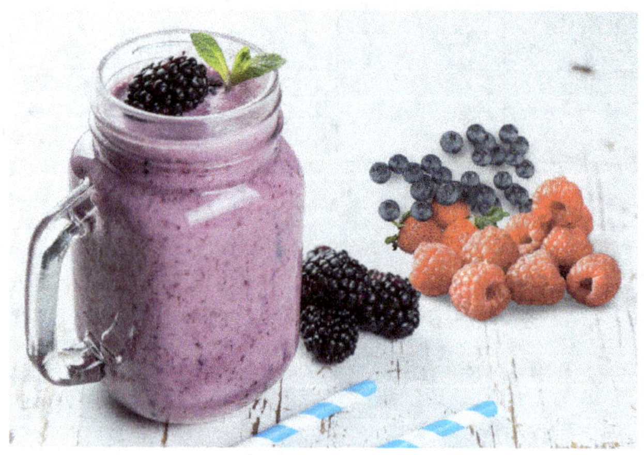

Nutritional Information (approx. per serving):

Calories	Carbohydrates	Protein	Fat
150	20g	8g	4g

Preparation:

1. In a blender, combine Greek yogurt, mixed berries, and honey (if desired).
2. Blend until smooth.
3. Pour into a glass and stir in chia seeds.

Green Apple Cinnamon Yogurt Blend

Ingredients:

- 1/2 cup Greek yogurt
- 1 small green apple, peeled and chopped
- 1/2 teaspoon ground cinnamon
- 1 tablespoon almond butter

Nutritional Information (approx. per serving):

Calories	Carbohydrates	Protein	Fat

180	22g	9g	6g

Preparation:

1. Blend Greek yogurt, chopped green apple, ground cinnamon, and almond butter until creamy.

2. Adjust thickness with a bit of water if needed.

Mango Coconut Yogurt Blend

Ingredients:

- 1/2 cup Greek yogurt
- 1/2 cup chopped fresh mango
- 2 tablespoons unsweetened coconut flakes
- 1/4 teaspoon vanilla extract

Nutritional Information (approx. per serving):

Calories	Carbohydrates	Protein	Fat

180	22g	9g	6g

Preparation:

1. Blend Greek yogurt, fresh mango, coconut flakes, and vanilla extract until smooth.
2. Adjust thickness by adding more yogurt if necessary.

Peach Ginger Yogurt Blend

Ingredients:

- 1/2 cup Greek yogurt
- 1 ripe peach, peeled and chopped
- 1/2 teaspoon grated fresh ginger
- 1 tablespoon honey (optional)

Nutritional Information (approx. per serving):

Calories	Carbohydrates	Protein	Fat

160	20g	9g	4g

Preparation:

1. Blend Greek yogurt, chopped ripe peach, fresh ginger, and honey (if desired) until well blended.

2. Add a few ice cubes for a colder blend.

Avocado Kiwi Yogurt Blend

Ingredients:

- 1/2 cup Greek yogurt
- 1 ripe avocado
- 1 ripe kiwi, peeled and chopped
- 1 tablespoon lime juice

Nutritional Information (approx. per serving):

Calories	Carbohydrates	Protein	Fat
190	20g	9g	7g

Preparation:

1. Blend Greek yogurt, ripe avocado, chopped kiwi, and lime juice until creamy.

2. Adjust the thickness by adding more yogurt if needed.

Low-Fat Milkshake Options

Vanilla Almond Milkshake

Ingredients:

- 1 cup low-fat milk (1%)
- 1/2 teaspoon almond extract
- 1/4 teaspoon ground cinnamon
- 1 tablespoon honey (optional)
- 1/2 cup ice cubes

Nutritional Information (approx. per serving):

Calories	Carbohydrates	Protein	Fat

| 120 | 14g | 8g | 3g |

Preparation:

- Blend low-fat milk, almond extract, ground cinnamon, honey (if using), and ice cubes until smooth.
- Pour into a glass and serve.

Coffee and Oat Milkshake

Ingredients:

- 1/2 cup brewed coffee (cooled)
- 1 cup low-fat oat milk
- 1 tablespoon unsweetened cocoa powder
- 1 tablespoon honey (optional)

Nutritional Information (approx. per serving):

Calories	Carbohydrates	Protein	Fat
110	20g	5g	2g

Preparation:

1. In a blender, combine cooled coffee, low-fat oat milk, cocoa powder, and honey (if desired).
2. Blend until frothy and well mixed.
3. Serve immediately.

Mango Turmeric Milkshake

Ingredients:

- 1 ripe mango, peeled and chopped
- 1 cup low-fat milk (1%)
- 1/2 teaspoon ground turmeric
- 1 tablespoon honey (optional)

Nutritional Information (approx. per serving):

Calories	Carbohydrates	Protein	Fat
170	30g	6g	2g

Preparation:

1. Blend ripe mango, low-fat milk, ground turmeric, and honey (if desired) until creamy.

2. Serve immediately.

Peanut Butter Chocolate Milkshake

Ingredients:

- 1 cup low-fat chocolate milk
- 1 tablespoon natural peanut butter
- 1/2 banana
- 1/4 cup low-fat Greek yogurt

Nutritional Information (approx. per serving):

Calories	Carbohydrates	Protein	Fat
220	30g	11g	6g

Preparation:

1. Blend low-fat chocolate milk, peanut butter, banana, and low-fat Greek yogurt until well combined.

2. Serve chilled.

Apple Cinnamon Oat Milkshake

Ingredients:

- 1/2 cup unsweetened applesauce
- 1 cup low-fat oat milk
- 1/2 teaspoon ground cinnamon
- 1 tablespoon honey (optional)

Nutritional Information (approx. per serving):

Calories	Carbohydrates	Protein	Fat
140	30g	3g	2g

Preparation:

1. Blend unsweetened applesauce, low-fat oat milk, ground cinnamon, and honey (if using) until smooth.
2. Pour into a glass and serve.

Cream-based Soups (Strained Or Blended)

Creamy Tomato Basil Soup

Ingredients:

- 1 can (28 oz) crushed tomatoes
- 1 cup low-sodium vegetable or chicken broth
- 1/2 cup heavy cream or half-and-half
- 1 small onion, chopped
- 2 cloves garlic, minced
- 2 tablespoons olive oil
- 1/4 cup fresh basil leaves, chopped
- Salt and pepper to taste

Nutritional Information (approx. per serving):

Calories	Carbohydrates	Protein	Fat
180	14g	3g	14g

Preparation:

1. In a pot, heat olive oil over medium heat. Sauté chopped onions and garlic until softened.

2. Add the crushed tomatoes, broth, and bring to a gentle simmer for 15 minutes.

3. Using an immersion blender, puree the mixture until smooth.

4. Stir in the heavy cream, fresh basil, salt, and pepper. Simmer for an additional 5 minutes.

5. Adjust seasoning as needed. Serve hot.

Cream of Broccoli Soup

Ingredients:

- 2 cups broccoli florets
- 1 cup low-sodium vegetable or chicken broth
- 1 cup low-fat milk
- 1 tablespoon unsalted butter
- 1 small onion, chopped

- 2 cloves garlic, minced

- Salt and pepper to taste

Nutritional Information (approx. per serving):

Calories	Carbohydrates	Protein	Fat
120	14g	8g	4g

Preparation:

1. In a saucepan, melt butter over medium heat. Sauté chopped onions and garlic until translucent.

2. Add broccoli and broth. Simmer for 15-20 minutes until the broccoli is tender.

3. Using an immersion blender or regular blender, puree the mixture until smooth.

4. Pour the puree back into the pot, add low-fat milk, and warm the soup.

5. Season with salt and pepper. Serve hot.

Creamy Carrot Ginger Soup

Ingredients:

- 4 cups chopped carrots
- 1 small onion, chopped
- 2 cloves garlic, minced
- 1 tablespoon fresh ginger, grated
- 4 cups low-sodium vegetable or chicken broth
- 1/2 cup heavy cream or coconut cream
- 2 tablespoons olive oil
- Salt and pepper to taste

Nutritional Information (approx. per serving):

Calories	Carbohydrates	Protein	Fat
160	20g	3g	8g

Preparation:

1. In a large pot, heat olive oil over medium heat. Sauté chopped onions, garlic, and ginger until fragrant.

2. Add chopped carrots and broth. Simmer for 20-25 minutes until carrots are soft.

3. Using a blender, puree the mixture until smooth.

4. Return the puree to the pot, add heavy cream, and warm the soup gently.

5. Season with salt and pepper. Serve warm.

Creamy Butternut Squash Soup

Ingredients:

- 4 cups cubed butternut squash
- 1 small onion, chopped
- 2 cloves garlic, minced
- 4 cups low-sodium vegetable or chicken broth
- 1/2 cup heavy cream or coconut cream
- 2 tablespoons olive oil

- 1/2 teaspoon ground nutmeg

- Salt and pepper to taste

Nutritional Information (approx. per serving):

Calories	Carbohydrates	Protein	Fat
200	26g	3g	10g

Preparation:

1. In a pot, heat olive oil over medium heat. Sauté chopped onions and garlic until tender.

2. Add butternut squash, broth, and nutmeg. Simmer for 20-25 minutes until squash is soft.

3. Puree the mixture using a blender until smooth.

4. Return the puree to the pot, add heavy cream, and warm the soup gently.

5. Season with salt and pepper. Serve hot.

Cream of Asparagus Soup

Ingredients:

- 2 cups chopped asparagus
- 1 small onion, chopped
- 2 cloves garlic, minced
- 4 cups low-sodium vegetable or chicken broth
- 1/2 cup heavy cream or coconut cream
- 2 tablespoons olive oil
- Salt and pepper to taste

Nutritional Information (approx. per serving):

Calories	Carbohydrates	Protein	Fat
170	18g	4g	9g

Preparation:

1. In a pot, heat olive oil over medium heat. Sauté chopped onions and garlic until softened.

2. Add chopped asparagus and broth. Simmer for 15-20 minutes until the asparagus is tender.

3. Blend the mixture until smooth using a blender.

4. Return the puree to the pot, add heavy cream, and gently heat the soup.

5. Season with salt and pepper. Serve hot.

Creamy Potato Leek Soup

Ingredients:

- 2 cups chopped potatoes
- 1 leek, white and light green parts chopped
- 2 cloves garlic, minced
- 4 cups low-sodium vegetable or chicken broth
- 1/2 cup low-fat milk
- 2 tablespoons unsalted butter
- Salt and pepper to taste

Nutritional Information (approx. per serving):

Calories	Carbohydrates	Protein	Fat
150	20g	4g	6g

Preparation:

1. In a pot, melt butter over medium heat. Sauté chopped leeks and garlic until softened.
2. Add chopped potatoes and broth. Simmer for 20-25 minutes until potatoes are soft.
3. Blend the mixture until smooth using an immersion blender or regular blender.
4. Return the puree to the pot, add low-fat milk, and gently heat the soup.
5. Season with salt and pepper. Serve hot.

CHAPTER 4:

SOFT FOODS AND BLENDED MEALS

Creamy Vegetable Purees

Creamy Carrot Puree

Ingredients:

- 4 cups chopped carrots
- 1 cup low-sodium vegetable broth
- 1/2 cup low-fat milk or coconut milk
- 1 tablespoon unsalted butter
- Salt and pepper to taste

Nutritional Information (approx. per serving):

Calories	Carbohydrates	Protein	Fat
120	16g	3g	5g

Preparation:

1. In a pot, combine chopped carrots and vegetable broth. Bring to a simmer and cook until the carrots are tender.

2. Using a blender, puree the cooked carrots along with the broth until smooth.

3. Return the puree to the pot, add low-fat milk, and warm it gently.

4. Stir in unsalted butter, salt, and pepper. Serve warm.

Creamy Cauliflower Puree

Ingredients:

- 1 head cauliflower, chopped into florets
- 2 cloves garlic, minced
- 2 cups low-sodium vegetable broth
- 1/2 cup low-fat milk or coconut milk
- 1 tablespoon unsalted butter
- Salt and pepper to taste

Nutritional Information (approx. per serving):

Calories	Carbohydrates	Protein	Fat
110	14g	4g	5g

Preparation:

1. In a pot, combine cauliflower, garlic, and vegetable broth. Simmer until the cauliflower is soft.
2. Use a blender to puree the cooked cauliflower with the broth until smooth.
3. Return the puree to the pot, add low-fat milk, and gently warm the soup.
4. Stir in unsalted butter, salt, and pepper. Serve warm.

Creamy Sweet Potato Puree

Ingredients:

- 2 large sweet potatoes, peeled and cubed
- 1 small apple, peeled and chopped

- 2 cups low-sodium vegetable broth

- 1/2 cup low-fat milk or coconut milk

- 1 tablespoon unsalted butter

- Pinch of cinnamon (optional)

- Salt and pepper to taste

Nutritional Information (approx. per serving):

Calories	Carbohydrates	Protein	Fat
140	24g	3g	4g

Preparation:

1. In a pot, combine sweet potatoes, apple, and vegetable broth. Simmer until sweet potatoes are tender.

2. Use a blender to puree the cooked sweet potatoes, apple, and broth until smooth.

3. Return the puree to the pot, add low-fat milk, and gently warm the soup.

4. Stir in unsalted butter, cinnamon (if using), salt, and pepper. Serve warm.

Creamy Parsnip Puree

Ingredients:

- 4 cups chopped parsnips
- 1 small onion, chopped
- 2 cloves garlic, minced
- 2 cups low-sodium vegetable broth
- 1/2 cup low-fat milk or almond milk
- 1 tablespoon olive oil
- Salt and pepper to taste

Nutritional Information (approx. per serving):

Calories	Carbohydrates	Protein	Fat
130	20g	3g	4g

Preparation:

1. In a saucepan, heat olive oil over medium heat. Sauté chopped onions and garlic until softened.

2. Add chopped parsnips and vegetable broth. Simmer until parsnips are soft.

3. Using a blender, puree the cooked parsnips and broth until smooth.

4. Return the puree to the saucepan, add low-fat milk, and gently warm the soup.

5. Season with salt and pepper. Serve warm.

Creamy Beetroot Puree

Ingredients:

- 3 medium beetroots, peeled and chopped
- 1 small potato, peeled and chopped
- 2 cups low-sodium vegetable broth
- 1/2 cup low-fat milk or coconut milk
- 1 tablespoon unsalted butter
- Salt and pepper to taste

Nutritional Information (approx. per serving):

Calories	Carbohydrates	Protein	Fat
150	20g	4g	5g

Preparation:

1. In a pot, combine chopped beetroots, potato, and vegetable broth. Simmer until vegetables are tender.
2. Use a blender to puree the cooked beetroots, potato, and broth until smooth.
3. Return the puree to the pot, add low-fat milk, and gently heat the soup.
4. Stir in unsalted butter, salt, and pepper. Serve warm.

Creamy Pumpkin Puree

Ingredients:

- 2 cups pumpkin puree (canned or fresh)
- 1 small onion, chopped

- 2 cloves garlic, minced

- 2 cups low-sodium vegetable broth

- 1/2 cup low-fat milk or almond milk

- 1 tablespoon olive oil

- 1/4 teaspoon ground nutmeg

- Salt and pepper to taste

Nutritional Information (per serving):

Calories	Carbohydrates	Protein	Fat
120	18g	3g	4g

Preparation:

1. In a saucepan, heat olive oil over medium heat. Sauté chopped onions and garlic until tender.

2. Add pumpkin puree and vegetable broth. Simmer for 10-15 minutes.

3. Using a blender, puree the cooked pumpkin mixture until smooth.

4. Return the puree to the saucepan, add low-fat milk, nutmeg, and gently heat the soup.

5. Season with salt and pepper. Serve warm.

Soft Meats and Fish Dishes

Baked Lemon Herb Chicken

Ingredients:

- 2 boneless, skinless chicken breasts
- 2 tablespoons olive oil
- 1 lemon (juice and zest)
- 2 cloves garlic, minced
- 1 teaspoon dried thyme
- Salt and pepper to taste

Nutritional Information (per serving):

Calories	Carbohydrates	Protein	Fat
200	2g	25g	8g

Preparation:

1. Preheat the oven to 375°F (190°C).

2. In a bowl, mix olive oil, lemon juice, lemon zest, minced garlic, dried thyme, salt, and pepper.

3. Place the chicken breasts in a baking dish. Pour the prepared mixture over the chicken.

4. Bake for 25-30 minutes until the chicken is fully cooked. Check for an internal temperature of 165°F (74°C).

Tender Pot Roast

Ingredients:

- 2 pounds chuck roast
- 1 onion, chopped
- 2 cloves garlic, minced
- 2 carrots, sliced
- 2 cups beef broth
- 1 tablespoon olive oil

- 1 teaspoon dried rosemary

- Salt and pepper to taste

Nutritional Information (per serving):

Calories	Carbohydrates	Protein	Fat
280	5g	30g	15g

Preparation:

1. Preheat the oven to 300°F (150°C).

2. Heat olive oil in an oven-safe pot. Brown the chuck roast on all sides.

3. Add chopped onion, minced garlic, sliced carrots, beef broth, dried rosemary, salt, and pepper.

4. Cover and bake for 3-4 hours until the meat is tender and easily shreds with a fork.

Soft Fish Filet in Lemon Butter Sauce

Ingredients:

- 2 white fish filets (tilapia, cod, or sole)
- 2 tablespoons unsalted butter
- 1 lemon (juice and zest)
- 2 cloves garlic, minced
- 2 tablespoons chopped parsley
- Salt and pepper to taste

Nutritional Information (per serving):

Calories	Carbohydrates	Protein	Fat
180	3g	25g	8g

Preparation:

1. Preheat a non-stick skillet over medium heat.
2. Season fish filets with salt and pepper.
3. Melt butter in the skillet. Add minced garlic and cook for a minute.
4. Place the fish filets in the skillet. Cook for about 3-4 minutes per side until cooked through.

5. Add lemon juice, zest, and chopped parsley. Cook for an additional minute before serving.

Soft Turkey Meatballs

Ingredients:

- 1 pound ground turkey
- 1/4 cup breadcrumbs
- 1/4 cup grated Parmesan cheese
- 1 egg
- 2 cloves garlic, minced
- 1 tablespoon chopped parsley
- Salt and pepper to taste

Nutritional Information (per serving):

Calories	Carbohydrates	Protein	Fat
220	10g	20g	10g

Preparation:

1. Preheat the oven to 375°F (190°C).

2. In a bowl, combine ground turkey, breadcrumbs, Parmesan cheese, egg, minced garlic, chopped parsley, salt, and pepper.

3. Form the mixture into meatballs and place them on a baking sheet.

4. Bake for 20-25 minutes until the meatballs are fully cooked.

Soft Salmon Cakes

Ingredients:

- 2 cans (14 oz each) canned salmon, drained
- 1/4 cup mayonnaise
- 1/4 cup breadcrumbs
- 1 egg
- 2 tablespoons chopped dill
- 1 tablespoon olive oil
- Salt and pepper to taste

Nutritional Information (per serving):

Calories	Carbohydrates	Protein	Fat
240	10g	25g	12g

Preparation:

1. In a bowl, combine canned salmon, mayonnaise, breadcrumbs, egg, chopped dill, salt, and pepper.
2. Form the mixture into patties.
3. Heat olive oil in a skillet over medium heat. Cook the salmon cakes for about 4-5 minutes per side until golden and heated through.

Tender Beef Stew

Ingredients:

- 1 pound beef stew meat
- 2 carrots, sliced
- 2 potatoes, cubed
- 1 onion, chopped
- 2 cloves garlic, minced

- 2 cups beef broth

- 1 tablespoon tomato paste

- 1 tablespoon olive oil

- 1 teaspoon dried thyme

- Salt and pepper to taste

Nutritional Information (per serving):

Calories	Carbohydrates	Protein	Fat
280	20g	25g	12g

Preparation:

1. Heat olive oil in a pot over medium heat. Brown the beef stew meat.

2. Add chopped onion, minced garlic, sliced carrots, cubed potatoes, beef broth, tomato paste, dried thyme, salt, and pepper.

3. Cover and simmer for 1.5-2 hours until the meat is tender and the vegetables are soft.

Soft Shredded Chicken Tacos

Ingredients:

- 2 boneless, skinless chicken breasts
- 1 teaspoon chili powder
- 1 teaspoon cumin
- 1/2 teaspoon garlic powder
- 1/2 teaspoon onion powder
- Salt and pepper to taste

Nutritional Information (per serving):

Calories	Carbohydrates	Protein	Fat
190	2g	25g	4g

Preparation:

1. Preheat the oven to 375°F (190°C).
2. Mix chili powder, cumin, garlic powder, onion powder, salt, and pepper.
3. Rub the spice mixture onto the chicken breasts.

4. Bake for 25-30 minutes until the chicken is fully cooked. Shred the chicken using two forks.

Soft Baked Cod with Herbs

Ingredients:

- 2 cod fillets
- 2 tablespoons olive oil
- 1 lemon (juice and zest)
- 2 cloves garlic, minced
- 1 tablespoon chopped fresh herbs (parsley, dill, or basil)
- Salt and pepper to taste

Nutritional Information (per serving):

Calories	Carbohydrates	Protein	Fat
220	2g	25g	8g

Preparation:

1. Preheat the oven to 375°F (190°C).

2. Place cod fillets in a baking dish.

3. In a bowl, mix olive oil, lemon juice, lemon zest, minced garlic, chopped herbs, salt, and pepper.

4. Pour the mixture over the fish.

5. Bake for 15-20 minutes until the fish is cooked through and flakes easily.

Blended Grains and Legumes

Quinoa Red Lentil Soup

Ingredients:

- 1/2 cup quinoa
- 1/2 cup red lentils
- 4 cups low-sodium vegetable broth
- 1 onion, chopped
- 2 cloves garlic, minced
- 1 teaspoon cumin
- Salt and pepper to taste

Nutritional Information (per serving):

Calories	Carbohydrates	Protein	Fat
220	40g	12g	2g

Preparation:

1. In a pot, combine quinoa, red lentils, vegetable broth, chopped onion, minced garlic, cumin, salt, and pepper.
2. Bring to a boil, then reduce heat and simmer for 20-25 minutes until grains and lentils are soft.
3. Blend the mixture until smooth using an immersion blender or regular blender.
4. Serve warm.

Creamy Brown Rice and Chickpea Porridge

Ingredients:

- 1/2 cup brown rice
- 1/2 cup cooked chickpeas

- 3 cups water or low-sodium vegetable broth
- 1/2 teaspoon turmeric
- 1/4 teaspoon ground ginger
- Salt to taste

Nutritional Information (per serving):

Calories	Carbohydrates	Protein	Fat
240	45g	10g	2g

Preparation:

1. In a pot, combine brown rice, cooked chickpeas, water or vegetable broth, turmeric, ground ginger, and salt.
2. Simmer for 30-35 minutes until the rice and chickpeas are soft.
3. Blend the mixture until smooth using a hand blender or food processor.
4. Serve warm, adding more liquid if a thinner consistency is desired.

Split Pea and Barley Soup

Ingredients:

- 1/2 cup split peas
- 1/2 cup barley
- 4 cups low-sodium vegetable broth
- 1 carrot, chopped
- 1 celery stalk, chopped
- 1 onion, chopped
- 2 cloves garlic, minced
- 1 teaspoon dried thyme
- Salt and pepper to taste

Nutritional Information (per serving):

Calories	Carbohydrates	Protein	Fat
230	45g	8g	2g

Preparation:

1. In a pot, combine split peas, barley, vegetable broth, chopped carrot, celery,

onion, minced garlic, dried thyme, salt, and pepper.

2. Bring to a boil, then simmer for 40-45 minutes until peas and barley are tender.

3. Blend the mixture until smooth using a hand blender or regular blender.

4. Serve warm.

Millet and Black Bean Congee

Ingredients:

- 1/2 cup millet
- 1/2 cup cooked black beans
- 3 cups water or low-sodium vegctablc broth
- 1/2 teaspoon ground coriander
- 1/4 teaspoon ground cumin
- Salt to taste

Nutritional Information (per serving):

Calories	Carbohydrates	Protein	Fat

210	40g	9g	1g

Preparation:

1. In a pot, combine millet, cooked black beans, water or vegetable broth, ground coriander, ground cumin, and salt.

2. Simmer for 25-30 minutes until millet is soft.

3. Blend the mixture until smooth using a hand blender or food processor.

4. Serve warm, adjusting the consistency with additional liquid if necessary.

Sorghum and Green Pea Puree

Ingredients:

- 1/2 cup sorghum
- 1/2 cup green peas (fresh or frozen)
- 3 cups water or low-sodium vegetable broth
- 1 tablespoon olive oil

- 1 teaspoon dried basil

- Salt and pepper to taste

Nutritional Information (per serving):

Calories	Carbohydrates	Protein	Fat
240	45g	7g	3g

Preparation:

1. In a pot, combine sorghum, green peas, water or vegetable broth, olive oil, dried basil, salt, and pepper.

2. Simmer for 40-45 minutes until sorghum and peas are tender.

3. Blend the mixture until smooth using an immersion blender or regular blender.

4. Serve warm.

Soft Amaranth and Lentil Mash
Ingredients:

- 1/2 cup amaranth

- 1/2 cup cooked green or brown lentils

- 3 cups low-sodium vegetable broth

- 2 tablespoons chopped fresh parsley

- 1 tablespoon lemon juice

- Salt to taste

Nutritional Information (per serving):

Calories	Carbohydrates	Protein	Fat
220	40g	10g	2g

Preparation:

1. In a pot, combine amaranth, cooked lentils, vegetable broth, chopped parsley, lemon juice, and salt.

2. Bring to a boil, then reduce heat and simmer for 20-25 minutes until amaranth is soft.

3. Blend the mixture until smooth using an immersion blender or regular blender.

4. Serve warm.

Soft Buckwheat and Black Eyed Pea Porridge

Ingredients:

- 1/2 cup buckwheat groats
- 1/2 cup cooked black-eyed peas
- 3 cups water or low-sodium vegetable broth
- 1/2 teaspoon smoked paprika
- 1/4 teaspoon ground turmeric
- Salt to taste

Nutritional Information (per serving):

Calories	Carbohydrates	Protein	Fat
240	45g	8g	2g

Preparation:

1. In a pot, combine buckwheat, cooked black-eyed peas, water or vegetable

broth, smoked paprika, ground turmeric, and salt.

2. Simmer for 25-30 minutes until buckwheat is soft.

3. Blend the mixture until smooth using a hand blender or food processor.

4. Serve warm, adjusting the consistency with additional liquid if needed.

Soft Red Quinoa and Pinto Bean Mash

Ingredients:

- 1/2 cup red quinoa
- 1/2 cup cooked pinto beans
- 3 cups low-sodium vegetable broth
- 2 tablespoons chopped fresh cilantro
- 1 tablespoon lime juice
- Salt to taste

Nutritional Information (per serving):

Calories	Carbohydrates	Protein	Fat

230	40g	9g	2g

Preparation:

1. In a pot, combine red quinoa, cooked pinto beans, vegetable broth, chopped cilantro, lime juice, and salt.

2. Bring to a boil, then reduce heat and simmer for 20-25 minutes until quinoa is cooked and beans are soft.

3. Blend the mixture until smooth using an immersion blender or regular blender.

4. Serve warm.

Soft Farro and Kidney Bean Soup

Ingredients:

- 1/2 cup farro
- 1/2 cup cooked kidney beans
- 4 cups low-sodium vegetable broth
- 1 tomato, chopped
- 1 bell pepper, chopped

- 1 onion, chopped

- 2 cloves garlic, minced

- 1 teaspoon dried oregano

- Salt and pepper to taste

Nutritional Information (per serving):

Calories	Carbohydrates	Protein	Fat
240	45g	10g	1g

Preparation:

1. In a pot, combine farro, cooked kidney beans, vegetable broth, chopped tomato, bell pepper, onion, minced garlic, dried oregano, salt, and pepper.

2. Simmer for 40-45 minutes until farro is tender.

3. Blend the mixture until smooth using an immersion blender or regular blenderServe warm.

CHAPTER 5:

SMALL BITES AND BALANCED MEALS

Mini Portioned Protein Meals

Egg and Spinach Muffin Cups

Ingredients:

- 4 eggs

- 1 cup chopped spinach

- 1/4 cup diced bell peppers

- Salt and pepper to taste

Nutritional Information (per muffin cup):

Calories	Carbohydrates	Protein	Fat
70	2g	7g	4g

Preparation:

1. Preheat the oven to 350°F (175°C).

2. Whisk the eggs in a bowl and add chopped spinach, diced bell peppers, salt, and pepper.

3. Pour the mixture into a greased muffin tin.

4. Bake for 15-20 minutes until the muffin cups are firm and lightly browned.

Tuna and Avocado Lettuce Wraps

Ingredients:

- 1 can tuna, drained
- 1 ripe avocado, mashed
- Lettuce leaves
- Optional: diced onions, tomatoes, or seasoning

Nutritional Information (per wrap):

Calories	Carbohydrates	Protein	Fat
150	6g	15g	8g

Preparation:

1. In a bowl, mix drained tuna and mashed avocado.

2. Spoon the tuna and avocado mixture onto lettuce leaves.

3. Optionally add diced onions, tomatoes, or preferred seasoning.

4. Wrap the lettuce around the filling to form a wrap.

Grilled Lemon Herb Chicken Skewers

Ingredients:

- Chicken breast, cut into cubes
- Lemon juice
- Fresh herbs (such as thyme, rosemary, or parsley)
- Salt and pepper

Nutritional Information (per serving):

Calories	Carbohydrates	Protein	Fat

200	0g	25g	3g

Preparation:

1. Marinate chicken cubes in lemon juice, fresh herbs, salt, and pepper.

2. Skewer the marinated chicken and grill until fully cooked.

3. Serve the grilled chicken skewers.

Salmon Cucumber Bites

Ingredients:

- Smoked or grilled salmon, flaked

- English cucumber, sliced

- Optional: dill, cream cheese

Nutritional Information (per serving):

Calories	Carbohydrates	Protein	Fat
120	3g	15g	5g

Preparation:

1. Place a slice of cucumber on a plate.

2. Top each cucumber slice with flaked salmon.

3. Optionally garnish with dill or a small amount of cream cheese.

Beef and Bell Pepper Skewers

Ingredients:

- Lean beef cubes

- Bell peppers, cut into chunks

- Olive oil, garlic, seasoning

Nutritional Information (per serving):

Calories	Carbohydrates	Protein	Fat
200	3g	25g	5g

Preparation:

1. Marinate beef cubes in olive oil, garlic, and preferred seasoning.

2. Skewer the beef cubes alternating with chunks of bell peppers.

3. Grill until the beef is cooked to the desired level.

Quinoa and Black Bean Stuffed Bell Peppers

Ingredients:

- Cooked quinoa

- Cooked black beans

- Bell peppers, halved and deseeded

- Optional: seasoning, cheese

Nutritional Information (per serving):

Calories	Carbohydrates	Protein	Fat
150	20g	12g	4g

Preparation:

1. Mix cooked quinoa and black beans, adding preferred seasoning.

2. Stuff halved bell peppers with the quinoa
   and black bean mixture.

3. Optionally top with a sprinkle of cheese
   and bake until the peppers are tender.

Shrimp and Zucchini Noodles

Ingredients:

- Shrimp, peeled and deveined
- Zucchini, spiralized into noodles
- Olive oil, garlic, herbs

Nutritional Information (per serving):

Calories	Carbohydrates	Protein	Fat
100	8g	20g	3g

Preparation:

1. Sauté shrimp in olive oil, garlic, and
   preferred herbs until fully cooked.

2. Add zucchini noodles to the pan and
   cook until slightly tender.

3. Serve the shrimp over the zucchini noodles.

Creative Ways with Beans and Tofu

Crispy Baked Tofu Nuggets

Ingredients:

- 1 block firm tofu, pressed and cut into cubes
- 2 tablespoons cornstarch
- 1 tablespoon soy sauce
- 1 teaspoon garlic powder
- 1/2 teaspoon paprika
- Cooking spray

Nutritional Information (per serving):

Calories	Carbohydrates	Protein	Fat
180	12g	12g	8g

Preparation:

1. Preheat the oven to 400°F (200°C).

2. Toss tofu cubes with cornstarch, soy sauce, garlic powder, and paprika until coated.

3. Place tofu on a baking sheet lined with parchment paper. Lightly spray the tofu with cooking spray.

4. Bake for 25-30 minutes, turning halfway through until crispy.

Mashed White Beans with Herbs

Ingredients:

- 1 can white beans, drained and rinsed
- 2 tablespoons olive oil
- 1 tablespoon chopped fresh rosemary
- 1 tablespoon chopped fresh thyme
- Salt and pepper to taste

Nutritional Information (per serving):

Calories	Carbohydrates	Protein	Fat

150	20g	8g	5g

Preparation:

1. In a bowl, mash white beans using a fork or potato masher.

2. Stir in olive oil, chopped rosemary, chopped thyme, salt, and pepper.

3. Mix until well combined and serve warm.

Black Bean and Tofu Scramble

Ingredients:

- 1 block firm tofu, crumbled
- 1 can black beans, drained and rinsed
- 1 red bell pepper, chopped
- 1 teaspoon cumin
- 1/2 teaspoon chili powder
- Salt and pepper to taste

Nutritional Information (per serving):

Calories	Carbohydrates	Protein	Fat
220	20g	15g	8g

Preparation:

1. In a skillet, sauté crumbled tofu, black beans, chopped red bell pepper, cumin, and chili powder until heated through.

2. Season with salt and pepper. Serve warm.

Tofu and Black-Eyed Pea Salad

Ingredients:

- 1 block firm tofu, diced
- 1 can black-eyed peas, drained and rinsed
- 1 cucumber, diced
- 2 tablespoons lemon juice
- 2 tablespoons olive oil
- 1 tablespoon chopped fresh parsley
- Salt and pepper to taste

Nutritional Information (per serving):

Calories	Carbohydrates	Protein	Fat
190	15g	12g	8g

Preparation:

1. In a bowl, combine diced tofu, black-eyed peas, diced cucumber, lemon juice, olive oil, chopped parsley, salt, and pepper.
2. Toss gently to mix. Serve chilled.

Tofu and Edamame Stir-Fry

Ingredients:

- 1 block firm tofu, cubed
- 1 cup shelled edamame
- 1 cup broccoli florets
- 2 tablespoons soy sauce
- 1 tablespoon sesame oil
- 1 teaspoon grated ginger

- 2 cloves garlic, minced

Nutritional Information (per serving):

Calories	Carbohydrates	Protein	Fat
220	18g	15g	10g

Preparation:

1. In a skillet, sauté cubed tofu, shelled edamame, and broccoli florets until slightly browned.
2. In a bowl, mix soy sauce, sesame oil, grated ginger, and minced garlic.
3. Pour the sauce over the tofu and vegetables. Stir-fry for a few minutes. Serve warm.

Balanced Nutritional Plates

Grilled Chicken with Quinoa and Roasted Vegetables

Ingredients:

- Grilled chicken breast
- 1/2 cup cooked quinoa
- Assorted roasted vegetables (bell peppers, zucchini, carrots)
- Mixed greens salad with a light vinaigrette

Nutritional Information:

Calories	Carbohydrates	Protein	Fat
350	25g	30g	15g

Preparation:

1. Grill the chicken breast until fully cooked.
2. Cook quinoa according to package instructions.
3. Roast assorted vegetables with a drizzle of olive oil at 400°F (200°C) until tender.

4. Assemble the plate with grilled chicken, a portion of quinoa, roasted vegetables, and a side of mixed greens with a light vinaigrette.

Salmon with Sweet Potato and Steamed Broccoli

Ingredients:

- Baked or grilled salmon fillet
- 1 small baked sweet potato
- Steamed broccoli florets
- Side salad with lemon dressing

Nutritional Information:

Calories	Carbohydrates	Protein	Fat
400	25g	25g	15g

Preparation:

1. Bake or grill the salmon fillet until fully cooked.

2. Bake a small sweet potato until tender.

3. Steam broccoli florets until they reach desired tenderness.

4. Arrange the plate with the salmon, baked sweet potato, steamed broccoli, and a side salad with a light lemon dressing.

Tofu Stir-Fry with Brown Rice and Mixed Vegetables

Ingredients:

- Stir-fried tofu cubes in a light sauce (low-sodium soy sauce, garlic, ginger)
- 1/2 cup cooked brown rice
- Stir-fried mixed vegetables (bell peppers, snap peas, carrots)
- Side of sliced fruit (pineapple or berries)

Nutritional Information:

Calories	Carbohydrates	Protein	Fat
300	35g	25g	10g

Preparation:

1. Stir-fry tofu cubes in a light sauce made of low-sodium soy sauce, garlic, and ginger until heated through.

2. Cook brown rice according to package instructions.

3. Stir-fry mixed vegetables in a non-stick pan until tender-crisp.

4. Plate the stir-fried tofu, brown rice, mixed vegetables, and a side of sliced fruit.

Turkey Chili with Whole Grain Bread and Side Salad

Ingredients:

- Homemade turkey chili (lean ground turkey, beans, tomatoes, onions, spices)
- 1-2 slices of whole grain bread
- Side salad with a light vinaigrette

Nutritional Information:

Calories	Carbohydrates	Protein	Fat
350	30g	25g	15g

Preparation:

1. Prepare turkey chili by cooking lean ground turkey with beans, tomatoes, onions, and preferred spices.
2. Toast whole grain bread slices.
3. Create a side salad with your choice of greens and a light vinaigrette.
4. Serve the turkey chili with a side of whole grain bread and the side salad.

Egg Omelette with Spinach, Whole Grain Toast, and Fruit

Ingredients:

- Spinach and mushroom omelette (made with egg whites or whole eggs)
- 1-2 slices of whole grain toast

- Sliced fruit (such as berries or melon)

Nutritional Information:

Calories	Carbohydrates	Protein	Fat
300	25g	20g	15g

Preparation:

1. Prepare an omelette with spinach and mushrooms using egg whites or whole eggs.
2. Toast whole grain bread slices.
3. Serve the omelette with whole grain toast and a side of sliced fruit.

Lentil Soup with Whole Grain Crackers and Greek Yogurt

Ingredients:

- Homemade lentil soup (made with lentils, vegetables, and spices)
- Whole grain crackers or breadsticks

- Greek yogurt with a drizzle of honey (if desired)

Nutritional Information:

Calories	Carbohydrates	Protein	Fat
250	30g	15g	10g

Preparation:

1. Prepare homemade lentil soup using lentils, vegetables, and preferred spices.
2. Serve the lentil soup with a side of whole grain crackers or breadsticks.
3. Accompany the meal with a serving of Greek yogurt and a drizzle of honey if desired.

Grilled Shrimp with Quinoa Salad and Steamed Asparagus

Ingredients:

- Grilled shrimp skewers or a fillet

- Quinoa salad (quinoa, cherry tomatoes, cucumber, herbs)
- Steamed asparagus spears

Nutritional Information:

Calories	Carbohydrates	Protein	Fat
350	30g	25g	15g

Preparation:

1. Grill shrimp skewers or a fillet until fully cooked.
2. Prepare a quinoa salad with cherry tomatoes, cucumber, and fresh herbs.
3. Steam asparagus until tender.
4. Serve the grilled shrimp with the quinoa salad and steamed asparagus.

Bean and Avocado Wrap with Side of Carrot Sticks and Hummus

Ingredients:

- Bean and avocado whole grain wrap
- Carrot sticks
- Hummus for dipping

Nutritional Information:

Calories	Carbohydrates	Protein	Fat
300	35g	15g	15g

Preparation:

1. Prepare a bean and avocado whole grain wrap with your choice of beans, avocado, vegetables, and whole grain wrap.
2. Slice carrots into sticks for a side.
3. Serve the wrap with carrot sticks and a side of hummus for dipping.

CHAPTER 6:

SNACKS AND TREATS

Nutrient-Dense Snack Ideas

Cottage Cheese and Pineapple Cubes

Ingredients:

- Low-fat cottage cheese

- Fresh pineapple, cubed

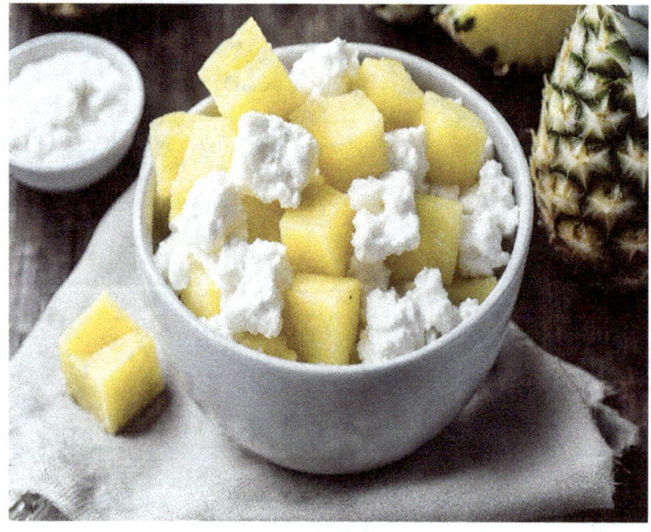

Nutritional Information:

Calories	Carbohydrates	Protein	Fat
150	15g	15g	5g

Preparation:

1. Serve a portion of low-fat cottage cheese with cubes of fresh pineapple.

Almond Butter with Apple Slices

Ingredients:

- Natural almond butter
- Apple, sliced

Nutritional Information:

Calories	Carbohydrates	Protein	Fat
200	20g	6g	12g

Preparation:

1. Dip apple slices into natural almond butter for a nutrient-rich snack.

Hard-Boiled Eggs with Hummus

Ingredients:

- Hard-boiled eggs
- Hummus

Nutritional Information:

Calories	Carbohydrates	Protein	Fat
150	8g	15g	10g

Preparation:

1. Enjoy hard-boiled eggs with a side of hummus for added flavor.

Tuna Salad on Whole Grain Crackers

Ingredients:

- Canned tuna
- Low-fat mayonnaise
- Diced celery
- Whole grain crackers

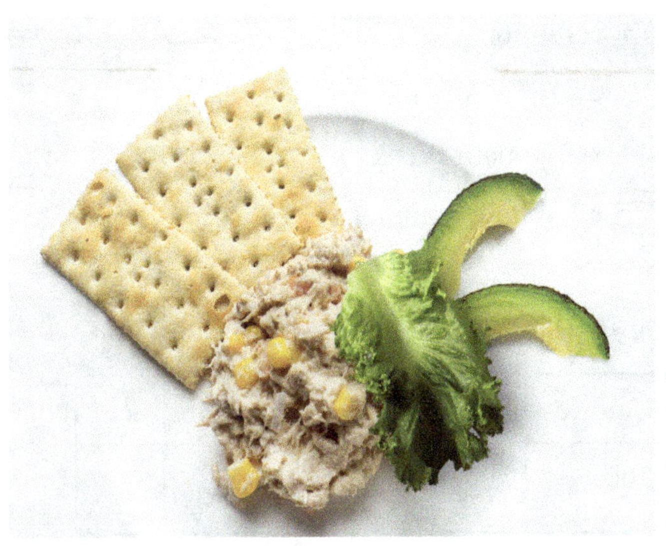

Nutritional Information:

Calories	Carbohydrates	Protein	Fat
200	15g	15g	6g

Preparation:

1. Prepare a simple tuna salad with low-fat mayonnaise and diced celery.

2. Serve the tuna salad on top of whole grain crackers for a satisfying snack.

Avocado and Tomato Toast

Ingredients:

- Ripe avocado
- Tomato slices
- Whole grain toast

Nutritional Information:

Calories	Carbohydrates	Protein	Fat
200	20g	6g	8g

Preparation:

1. Mash ripe avocado and spread it over whole grain toast.
2. Top with slices of tomato for a nutrient-packed snack.

Roasted Chickpeas

Ingredients:

- Canned chickpeas
- Olive oil, spices

Nutritional Information:

Calories	Carbohydrates	Protein	Fat
200	25g	8g	8g

Preparation:

1. Drain and rinse canned chickpeas, toss with olive oil and preferred spices.

2. Roast in the oven until crispy for a nutrient-rich and crunchy snack.

Sugar-Free Dessert Delights

Berries and Cream

Ingredients:

- Mixed berries (strawberries, blueberries, raspberries)
- Unsweetened whipped cream or Greek yogurt

Nutritional Information:

Calories	Carbohydrates	Protein	Fat

100	10g	4g	4g

Preparation:

1. Wash and dry a variety of fresh berries.

2. Serve the mixed berries with a dollop of unsweetened whipped cream or Greek yogurt.

Avocado Chocolate Mousse

Ingredients:

- Ripe avocados
- Unsweetened cocoa powder
- Unsweetened almond milk
- Stevia or another sugar substitute

Nutritional Information:

Calories	Carbohydrates	Protein	Fat
150	10g	2g	8g

Preparation:

1. Blend ripe avocados, unsweetened cocoa powder, unsweetened almond milk, and a sugar substitute until smooth.

2. Chill the mixture in the refrigerator before serving.

Baked Apples with Cinnamon

Ingredients:

- Apples, cored and sliced
- Ground cinnamon

Nutritional Information:

Calories	Carbohydrates	Protein	Fat
100	15g	1g	0.5g

Preparation:

1. Place sliced apples on a baking sheet and sprinkle with ground cinnamon.

2. Bake until the apples are soft and slightly caramelized.

Yogurt Bark

Ingredients:

- Unsweetened Greek yogurt
- Sugar-free nuts or seeds (like chopped almonds, pumpkin seeds)
- Sugar-free dried fruits (like cranberries or apricots)

Nutritional Information:

Calories	Carbohydrates	Protein	Fat
150	12g	8g	6g

Preparation:

1. Spread unsweetened Greek yogurt on a baking sheet.
2. Sprinkle with sugar-free nuts, seeds, and dried fruits.
3. Freeze until firm, then break into pieces for a yogurt bark snack.

Coconut Almond Bites

Ingredients:

- Unsweetened shredded coconut

- Almond flour

- Almond extract

- Unsweetened coconut milk

- Stevia or sugar substitute

Nutritional Information:

Calories	Carbohydrates	Protein	Fat
120	8g	4g	8g

Preparation:

1. Combine unsweetened shredded coconut, almond flour, almond extract, unsweetened coconut milk, and a sugar substitute.

2. Form into small bites and refrigerate until set.

Protein-Packed Frozen Yogurt Bites

Ingredients:

- Unsweetened Greek yogurt
- Sugar-free protein powder
- Stevia or another sugar substitute
- Mixed berries (optional)

Nutritional Information:

Calories	Carbohydrates	Protein	Fat
100	8g	10g	4g

Preparation:

1. Mix unsweetened Greek yogurt with sugar-free protein powder and a sugar substitute.
2. Spoon the mixture into small bite-sized molds, optionally adding mixed berries.
3. Freeze until set, then enjoy as a frozen treat.

CHAPTER 7:

28 DAYS (4 WEEKS) MEAL PLAN

Meal Plan Week 1: Clear Liquid Diet

Day 1

Breakfast: Clear vegetable or chicken broth

Snack: Sugar-free gelatin (clear)

Lunch: Plain chicken or vegetable broth

Snack: Popsicles (sugar-free and clear)

Dinner: Clear beef or fish broth

Day 2

Breakfast: Sugar-free fruit juice (diluted)

Snack: Clear vegetable or chicken broth

Lunch: Clear, strained vegetable or chicken broth

Snack: Clear fruit juice (diluted)

Dinner: Sugar-free gelatin (clear)

Day 3

Breakfast: Clear protein drink (check with your healthcare provider for suitable options)

Snack: Clear beef or chicken broth

Lunch: Strained chicken or vegetable broth

Snack: Popsicles (sugar-free and clear)

Dinner: Clear fish or vegetable broth

Day 4

Breakfast: Clear protein drink

Snack: Sugar-free gelatin (clear)

Lunch: Clear beef or chicken broth

Snack: Clear vegetable or fish broth

Dinner: Clear strained vegetable or chicken broth

Day 5

Breakfast: Sugar-free fruit juice (diluted)

Snack: Clear vegetable or chicken broth

Lunch: Clear fish or beef broth

Snack: Sugar-free gelatin (clear)

Dinner: Clear strained vegetable or chicken broth

Day 6

Breakfast: Clear protein drink

Snack: Sugar-free gelatin (clear)

Lunch: Strained chicken or vegetable broth

Snack: Clear vegetable or fish broth

Dinner: Clear beef or chicken broth

Day 7

Breakfast: Sugar-free fruit juice (diluted)

Snack: Clear vegetable or chicken broth

Lunch: Clear fish or beef broth

Snack: Sugar-free gelatin (clear)

Dinner: Clear strained vegetable or chicken broth

Meal Plan Week 2: Full Liquid Pureed Diet

Day 1

Breakfast: Protein shake (low sugar, blended with water or a non-dairy milk alternative)

Snack: Blended low-fat yogurt or cottage cheese

Lunch: Pureed vegetable soup (broth-based)

Snack: Fruit smoothie (blended with low-fat yogurt and a small amount of fruit)

Dinner: Blended chicken or fish with broth for a pureed protein meal

Day 2

Breakfast: Protein shake (blended with water or a non-dairy milk alternative)

Snack: Blended low-fat cottage cheese or yogurt

Lunch: Pureed split pea or lentil soup

Snack: Fruit or vegetable smoothie (low sugar, with added protein if desired)

Dinner: Pureed beef or vegetable stew

Day 3

Breakfast: Protein shake (blended with water or a non-dairy milk alternative)

Snack: Blended low-fat yogurt or cottage cheese

Lunch: Pureed chicken or vegetable soup

Snack: Fruit smoothie (with added protein if desired)

Dinner: Pureed fish or bean soup

Day 4

Breakfast: Protein shake (blended with water or a non-dairy milk alternative)

Snack: Blended low-fat cottage cheese or yogurt

Lunch: Pureed broccoli or cauliflower soup

Snack: Fruit or vegetable smoothie (low sugar, with added protein if desired)

Dinner: Pureed turkey or vegetable stew

Day 5

Breakfast: Protein shake (blended with water or a non-dairy milk alternative)

Snack: Blended low-fat yogurt or cottage cheese

Lunch: Pureed spinach or asparagus soup

Snack: Fruit smoothie (with added protein if desired)

Dinner: Pureed ham or mixed vegetable soup

Day 6

Breakfast: Protein shake (blended with water or a non-dairy milk alternative)

Snack: Blended low-fat cottage cheese or yogurt

Lunch: Pureed chicken or tomato soup

Snack: Fruit or vegetable smoothie (low sugar, with added protein if desired)

Dinner: Pureed fish or bean stew

Day 7

Breakfast: Protein shake (blended with water or a non-dairy milk alternative)

Snack: Blended low-fat yogurt or cottage cheese

Lunch: Pureed vegetable or chicken soup

Snack: Fruit smoothie (with added protein if desired)

Dinner: Pureed beef or vegetable stew

Meal Plan Week 3: Soft Foods And Blended Meals

Day 1

Breakfast: Scrambled eggs (soft and well-cooked)

Snack: Greek yogurt (plain or flavored, low in sugar)

Lunch: Mashed sweet potatoes or butternut squash

Snack: Applesauce or blended pear

Dinner: Pureed chicken or fish

Day 2

Breakfast: Cottage cheese (low-fat)

Snack: Blended banana or mango

Lunch: Creamy vegetable soup (well-blended)

Snack: Pureed avocado or guacamole

Dinner: Soft-cooked ground turkey or tofu

Day 3

Breakfast: Oatmeal (cooked to a soft consistency)

Snack: Blended low-fat ricotta cheese

Lunch: Pureed vegetable and bean chili

Snack: Pureed melon or berries

Dinner: Mashed beans or lentils

Day 4

Breakfast: Scrambled eggs with finely chopped spinach

Snack: Blended peach or nectarine

Lunch: Pureed broccoli or cauliflower soup

Snack: Pureed pear or applesauce

Dinner: Soft-cooked ground chicken or beef

Day 5

Breakfast: Cottage cheese (low-fat)

Snack: Blended banana or mango

Lunch: Creamy vegetable and chicken soup (well-blended)

Snack: Pureed avocado or guacamole

Dinner: Soft-cooked ground turkey or tofu

Day 6

Breakfast: Oatmeal (cooked to a soft consistency)

Snack: Blended low-fat ricotta cheese

Lunch: Mashed sweet potatoes or butternut squash

Snack: Pureed melon or berries

Dinner: Mashed beans or lentils

Day 7

Breakfast: Scrambled eggs (soft and well-cooked)

Snack: Greek yogurt (plain or flavored, low in sugar)

Lunch: Pureed vegetable and bean chili

Snack: Pureed pear or applesauce

Dinner: Soft-cooked ground chicken or beef

Meal Plan Week 4: Pureed + Soft Diet

Day 1

Breakfast: Blended oatmeal with mashed bananas

Snack: Pureed cottage cheese

Lunch: Mashed sweet potatoes

Snack: Blended peaches or pears

Dinner: Pureed chicken or fish with well-cooked vegetables

Day 2

Breakfast: Scrambled eggs (soft and well-cooked)

Snack: Pureed low-fat Greek yogurt

Lunch: Blended vegetable soup

Snack: Applesauce or blended berries

Dinner: Soft-cooked ground turkey or tofu

Day 3

Breakfast: Pureed avocado or guacamole

Snack: Blended oatmeal with mashed berries

Lunch: Pureed broccoli or cauliflower soup

Snack: Pureed cottage cheese

Dinner: Mashed beans or lentils

Day 4

Breakfast: Blended peach or nectarine with low-fat yogurt

Snack: Soft-cooked scrambled eggs with finely chopped spinach

Lunch: Pureed vegetable and chicken soup

Snack: Blended pear or applesauce

Dinner: Soft-cooked ground chicken or beef

Day 5

Breakfast: Oatmeal (cooked to a soft consistency) with mashed bananas

Snack: Pureed low-fat Greek yogurt

Lunch: Mashed sweet potatoes

Snack: Blended peaches or pears

Dinner: Pureed fish or chicken with well-cooked vegetables

Day 6

Breakfast: Scrambled eggs (soft and well-cooked)

Snack: Blended cottage cheese

Lunch: Blended vegetable soup

Snack: Applesauce or blended berries

Dinner: Soft-cooked ground turkey or tofu

Day 7

Breakfast: Pureed avocado or guacamole

Snack: Blended oatmeal with mashed berries

Lunch: Pureed broccoli or cauliflower soup

Snack: Pureed low-fat Greek yogurt

Dinner: Mashed beans or lentils

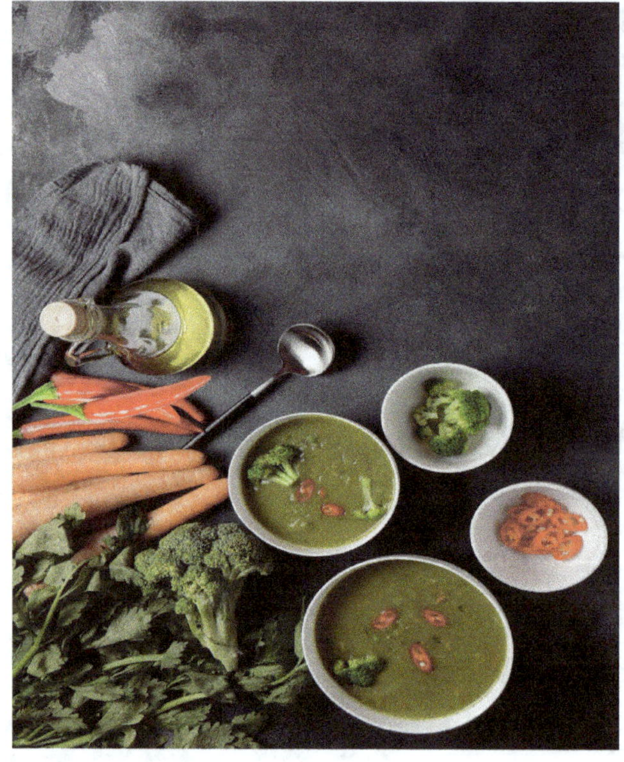

☐ Dear readers of the Gastric Sleeve Bariatric Cookbook, your feedback is invaluable! Have you explored the delicious, health-conscious recipes and insightful tips tailored to support your post-surgery journey? Your review can help others discover the nourishing and flavorful options this cookbook offers. Share your thoughts on how the recipes have contributed to your recovery, health, and newfound culinary adventures. Your review might be the encouragement someone seeks to embark on their own bariatric journey with confidence. Take a moment to reflect on your experience and leave a review for the Gastric Sleeve Bariatric Cookbook. Your words can guide and inspire others on their path to a healthier lifestyle. Thank you for being a part of this transformative journey! □□

CHAPTER 8:

CONCLUSION

Mindful Eating Practices

1. **Chew Thoroughly:** After gastric sleeve surgery, it's essential to chew food slowly and thoroughly. Aim for at least 20-30 chews per bite. This aids in digestion and prevents discomfort.

2. **Focus on Nutrient-Dense Foods:** Prioritize nutrient-dense foods such as lean protein, vegetables, fruits, and whole grains. These choices provide essential nutrients without excess calories.

3. **Smaller, Frequent Meals:** Consume smaller portions spread throughout the day. Dividing meals into 4-6 smaller portions can help manage hunger and prevent overeating.

4. **Mindful Portion Control:** Use smaller plates or containers to help manage portion sizes. Being mindful of portion control is crucial for managing weight and preventing discomfort.

5. **Eat Without Distractions:** Avoid eating in front of screens or while working. Focus on the meal, savoring each bite, and paying attention to feelings of fullness.

6. **Stay Hydrated:** Drink water between meals to stay hydrated. However, avoid drinking during meals, as it can cause discomfort and lead to feeling full too quickly.

7. **Identify Hunger and Fullness Signals:** Learn to recognize your body's signals for hunger and fullness. Eat slowly and pause between bites to assess how full you feel. Stop eating when you feel satisfied.

8. **Avoid Carbonated Beverages and Straws:** These can introduce excess air into your digestive system, potentially causing discomfort or bloating.

9. **Practice Mindfulness Techniques:** Incorporate mindfulness or relaxation techniques before eating to help reduce stress and promote mindful eating. This can include deep breathing, meditation, or simply taking a moment to appreciate your meal.

10. **Seek Support and Guidance:** Join support groups or work with a dietitian or counselor experienced in post-gastric sleeve surgery nutrition. They can provide guidance, support, and helpful tips for long-term success.

Incorporating Exercise into a New Lifestyle

1. **Start Slowly:** Begin with low-impact exercises such as walking, swimming, or cycling. Gradually increase intensity and duration as your body adjusts.

2. **Consult Your Doctor:** Before starting any exercise program, consult your healthcare provider or a fitness professional to determine a safe and suitable regimen based on your individual health and recovery.

3. **Consistency Over Intensity:** Focus on consistency rather than intense workouts. Regular, moderate exercise is more important than occasional intense sessions. Aim for at least 30 minutes of activity most days of the week.

4. **Strength Training:** Incorporate resistance training to build and maintain

muscle mass. This can include bodyweight exercises, resistance bands, or light weights. Strong muscles can help with metabolism and overall strength.

5. **Listen to Your Body:** Pay attention to your body's signals. If you experience pain, dizziness, or discomfort during exercise, stop and consult your doctor. It's important to exercise safely.

6. **Set Realistic Goals:** Establish achievable short-term and long-term goals. This could be as simple as increasing daily steps or aiming to exercise a certain number of times per week.

7. **Enjoy Varied Activities:** Mix up your workouts to prevent boredom and work different muscle groups. Try activities like yoga, dancing, or even gardening. Enjoyable activities make it easier to stick to an exercise routine.

8. **Stay Hydrated:** Drink water before, during, and after exercising to stay hydrated, especially considering the reduced stomach capacity after surgery.

9. **Use Support Systems:** Consider joining exercise groups, working out with a friend, or seeking guidance from a fitness trainer or physical therapist. Support and guidance can help keep you motivated and ensure proper form.

10. **Track Progress:** Keep a record of your exercises, noting improvements and milestones. This can help maintain motivation and provide a sense of accomplishment.

Handling Challenges and Maintaining Progress

1. **Support Network:** Build a strong support system. Connect with friends,

family, support groups, or online communities of individuals who have undergone similar surgeries. Sharing experiences and advice can be immensely helpful.

2. **Regular Follow-Ups:** Attend regular follow-up appointments with your healthcare team, including the surgeon, nutritionist, and psychologist if necessary. They can provide guidance, monitor progress, and address any concerns.

3. **Mindful Eating:** Practice mindful eating by focusing on the meal, chewing slowly, and stopping when you feel full.

4. **Healthy Food Choices:** Prioritize nutrient-dense foods, including lean protein, fruits, vegetables, and whole grains. Limit processed and high-calorie foods to support weight loss and overall health.

5. **Stay Active:** Maintain a regular exercise routine. Incorporate both aerobic exercises and strength training to support weight management and overall well-being.

6. **Celebrate Non-Scale Victories:** Progress isn't just about the number on the scale. Celebrate non-scale victories, such as increased energy, improved stamina, better fitting clothes, or achieving new fitness milestones.

7. **Mindset Shift:** Embrace a mindset shift. Focus on health improvements, increased mobility, and the positive impact on overall well-being rather than solely on the number of pounds lost.

8. **Manage Emotional Challenges:** Seek professional support if you're struggling with emotional challenges post-surgery. Therapy or counseling can help address

any underlying issues and develop coping strategies.

9. **Hydration and Vitamins:** Ensure adequate hydration and take required vitamins and supplements as recommended by your healthcare provider. This is crucial for supporting your overall health, especially after the surgery.

10. **Adapt to Changes:** Be adaptable and patient. Your body and lifestyle will evolve after surgery. Embrace these changes and find new, sustainable habits that work for you.

11. **Track Progress and Set Goals:** Keep a journal to track your progress, noting achievements and areas for improvement.

www.ingramcontent.com/pod-product-compliance
Lightning Source LLC
Chambersburg PA
CBHW070934260726
48661CB00003B/983